PARDON MY PSYCHOSIS

JAMES COAST

Printed in the United States of America.
For more information, please contact:
Email: jamesc@voicelesstovictory.org
www.voicelesstovictory.org
www.jamescoast.com

Cover design by Rafael Andres

Library of Congress Control Number: 2023922926
ISBN – Paperback 979-8-9892044-0-3
ISBN – Hardcover 979-8-9892044-1-0
ISBN – eBook 979-8-9892044-2-7
1st edition March 2024

This book is dedicated to my family and friends who surrounded me with love and support during the most confusing time of my life. Without each and every one of you, I would not be who I am today.

CHAPTER 1

A once-normal life now shattered like a piece of defective pottery at the hands of its distraught maker. How did I break so easily? Or better yet, why did I break so thoroughly? I'm sure those answers won't come this side of heaven, but knowing God is not the author of chaos, I can only hope to unravel the confusion that is now my life.

I've had a normal life for forty years. A loving wife of eighteen years, two wonderful children, and a yappy little dog. We were the type of family that comes with the frame, picture perfect. Now there I sat in a psychiatrist's office, pretending to listen as my eyes shifted from the floor to the photos of jazz legends lining the walls. Bipolar 1 with severe psychosis was the diagnosis. At that point, it didn't even register. Memories of the previous weeks were nothing more than broken bits and battered pieces. The doctor seemed amicable enough, though. His calm, compassionate speech and silver-ladened hair said more about his level of expertise than the degrees hanging behind his head.

For my wife, the diagnosis came as a relief. Sunken into the electric blue chair beside me, she finally had an answer for the chaos she endured on my behalf. Her heavy eyes and slouched shoulders reflected the aftermath of my psychotic break. On the other hand, I had no clue what was happening around me, and things weren't normal anymore. It would be weeks before I came to terms with what happened and how intense my erratic behavior had been toward my family and friends.

Was the combination of hallucinations and delusions the absolute truth of my experience? Were brain chemicals and environmental conditions truly responsible for launching me into an alternate reality that only existed in the theater of my mind? Or was there a chance spiritual warfare played a role in what the natural world considered my psychotic break?

To get there, I had to go back to when the boundaries

between reality, spirituality, and mania began melting together.

***

In the fall of 2021, I noticed my daughter's relationship with the Lord blossoming into a beautiful, fulfilling relationship. Mine paled in comparison, proving my role as head of household had been neglected. I knew it was time to step up, dive in, and pursue the Lord. What began as a twenty-minute Bible reading every night became hours of studying and video-watching. From midnight sermon marathons to before-dawn prayer sessions, seeking God's Word became all-consuming. Over the next few months, my relationship with God and the Holy Spirit deepened beyond any fathomable expectation.

Or so I thought. Now I'm left asking myself how the mania snuck in and consumed me with such stealth. This question still tugs at my soul. What I saw, heard, and felt bounced between a beautiful fairytale and the most heart-pounding nightmare imaginable. Mania is no respecter of persons, but it was the fuel for the wildest ride I've ever taken.

The usual eight o'clock bedtime crept closer to midnight with each passing week. This wouldn't have been an issue, but as the nights got later, the mornings came earlier. Running on God's time without sleep did not affect me. In fact, I felt better than I had in years. The words in the Bible came alive with each passing day. Each verse was like looking at a snowflake through a microscope: uniquely complex and independently beautiful. Opening the Bible was like free-falling from a plane over a snow-capped mountain. The speed and intensity of barreling toward the rocky cliffs matched the intensity of how I tried to discern the Scriptures.

Then it shook me. A wake-up call so profound my life would never be the same. It was my call to action. During one of my late-night sessions, a pastor referenced Revelation 21:8: "But the cowardly, the unbelieving, the vile, the murderers, the sexually immoral, those who practice magic arts, the idolaters, and all liars, they will be consigned to the fiery lake of burning sulfur. This is the second death" (NIV). The verse hit home and held on with no intention of letting go. The line heading straight to hell, with me leading the way, resonated like an old church bell on a quiet Sunday morning.

Baptized in my twenties, what had I done since to advance the kingdom of God? The "cowardly" at the head of the line was me. A believer, yes, but a believer who chose self and safety over the faith and the unknown it takes to follow Jesus. With newfound depth and understanding of Scripture, I knew the world's view wanted me to jump this line and run for a friendlier crowd to hang out with. This, however, was my line, and these were the same people Jesus himself came to break bread with and minister to. My job was to change the line's direction, not abandon the people. This verse, among others, would soon be used on friends and coworkers. I was on a mission to save them even if they didn't need it.

Every week at work we had what I call Prayer Meeting Mondays. It was an hour set aside when four of us gathered to pray and discuss company matters on a Christian level. This was the highlight of every week. Each Monday, one of us brought a verse or topic of discussion to lead the meeting. The Holy Spirit was connecting us on a higher level every week. Each added to what someone else brought for the day. Like a symphony, the verses were layered by someone else's commentary in the room. I would sit and

listen to all the beautiful Scripture and deep conversations.
Every time, without fail, I would jump in to add what I felt
was given to me by God himself. At first, nothing seemed
out of place to my coworkers. After all, we were in those
meetings to speak openly about God and what He was
doing in our lives and company.

Then Friday morning, April 8, rolled around with a
charge of electricity in the air. This was the first warning
sign of what was to come, but I was clueless. The snaking
country roads plotting the course to work were usually full
of headlights illuminating the way. Not this day, though.
The deserted roads, to me, symbolized the less-crowded
path Christians are called to walk. I hummed along to
the upbeat music and fine-tuned a prayer for my arrival
at work with ease. Reaching work, I parked and walked
through the dusty parking lot to the corner of the building.
Over time, I developed a morning routine of praying for
the business and the people while placing my hand on the
side of the building.

Admittingly, it is a sight not seen often. But with no
intention of fitting in, the rough textured block wall drew
my hand like a magnet. The prayers sometimes lasted for

seconds; other times, they went long enough for someone to raise an eyebrow. Occasionally, a passerby would stop and ask if I was okay while making their way down the stone pathway to the office doors.

The rumbling of diesel engines and heavy equipment played melodically in the background as the rising sun warmed the back of my neck. Most mornings, dust from the trucks coming and going filled the air thick enough to hide the fifteen-acre inventory lot behind the main office. Not that morning, however, as I saw the world crystal clear while turning the corner to walk inside and find my desk.

This Friday marked a solid torturous week of the building's metal roof being ripped off and replaced. It's a long building, and the progress was excruciatingly slow. They installed one new panel as each old one was pried from its resting place. The shuffling feet above my head was the first sign the crew had made it to my side of the building. The second was the pounding above my head for hours as dust fell from the ceiling tiles. The more they hammered, the more dust floated down from them until it was like a shaken snow globe.

An alarm sounded from deep in my gut. It was undeniable at the time. I knew this was no ordinary roof replacement. It was a spiritual attack on the company. I wasn't sure how long the ceiling would hold. All I knew was this was God's company, so I sprang into action. No one else knew the reality of what was happening. Of course, they couldn't; how could they see it for what it was? I was the one chosen to defend this place. They couldn't see in the Spirit like I could, because they wouldn't be able to handle it. Not wanting to draw attention, I strolled to the back door casually. There was no need to alarm anyone. I had everything under complete control.

Behind the office is a large metal warehouse where building products are stored out of the weather, with a bay door at each end. When it's sunny, the doors let in enough daylight to make out what's inside. My calm steps turned into a battle charge toward the closest bay door once outside where all the inbound freight collects. I knew it had to be the entry point for spirits to creep in, clinging to inventory. I knew I would be outnumbered with thousands of items, but if these spirits wanted to wage war, I was ready to give them one.

Entering the warehouse, I searched from one end to

the other like a detective searching for clues. I was shuffling through, on edge as if it were an abandoned house at midnight, taking note of each nook and cranny. Every dark place my enemy might be hiding was checked. To the ordinary eye, things appeared normal, but I knew something was in there. The weight of its presence was trying to overtake me. After a few times back and forth, I built enough courage and launched into prayer. I paced, from one end back to the other, my arms out, saying, "Come and get me." Reaching the pinnacle, I stopped in the center and lowered my head with closed eyes. This was it, the final push to cleanse the warehouse. Arms raised and prepared to launch into prayer, a tap on the shoulder sent me through the roof. "You okay?" asked the hesitant warehouse worker.

"I am now, buddy, and so are you." The warehouse was done, and it was time to take the battle to the rest of the property.

I climbed into my truck, realizing it was the safest place to be. I kept a Bible in the console, and praise music was all I listened to at the time. Everyone knows that crazy, loud praise music is the best way to overpower and run off any lingering spirits. The windows came down, and the volume cranked up. I'm not talking a touch above average volume, though. I'm talking soul-piercing, earth-trembling, stronghold-breaking decibels. The sound waves radiated outward like the ripples of an atomic bomb, sure to destroy all the evil spirits in its path.

As I pulled through the gate leading to the rest of the property, two cast stone lion heads mounted in the weathered stone walls jumped at me for the first time. One on each side of the entry. Their jagged teeth were exposed, and their snarling faces were frozen in eternal battle. I had worked there for years but never noticed these beasts guarding our entry gate. They were put there for a specific purpose, but why?

Meditating on it for a moment, my spirit made the connection. They face east in defiance of the rising sun. East and west have no endpoints. They are a continuous, never-ending loop. Throughout history, people have worshipped the sun. In our day and age, the sun's golden glow is replaced by the relentless pursuit of money. The lust for riches is no different from the sun's endless loop circling east to west.

The lions were mounted for such a time as this. They watched my back as I jumped faith-first into battle. Volume blaring, I cruised through the gate with my arm out of the window, raised toward the sky. Praise and prayer belted from the truck during three slow loops around the property. I wove in and out of delivery trucks and customer vehicles, making my presence known. They didn't know what I was doing, but this was how it had to be. I didn't mind the funny looks at the time. I thought most "normal" people would never know what I knew, and this level of spiritual warfare would break them.

I returned to my small, dull cubicle and sank back into being a run-of-the-mill office worker again. The pounding on the roof had subsided, and the thin layer of dust coating my keyboard was the sole trace of the war raging moments ago. No bodies to collect, no wounded soldiers to care for, no parade or celebration. Superheroes must feel the same way. Enthralled in a brutal war one minute, returning to emails and pencil-pushing moments later wasn't easy. This is what the prophets of the Bible must have endured.

I received the gift of peering through the fragile veil separating the spiritual realm and the world as most understand it. Being brand-new to this, I couldn't speak of it to anyone; they would think I was crazy. As I stood and packed it in for the day, it was the perfect chance to inspect the room. All clear. As I soaked in victory for one last second, I realized my desk faced west. I sat with my back to the east in defiance of the rising sun and never noticed.

After dinner that evening, my wife hit me with a long list of honey-dos. The way the list works at our house is each time a task is knocked off, another appears. This time, however, my negotiating skills were on point. She agreed nothing would be added to the list until everything was crossed off. It was evident God had my back and wanted me to focus on fine-tuning my spiritual gifts. It was the first negotiation I'd ever won with my wife, and the fact that these chores would take a while was fine. Ordinary people do them all the time, and I knew I could get them done much faster, being on God's time. After all, tomorrow was a new day with plenty of time for chores.

Sleep evaded me again that night. With headphones in, I tossed and turned to the soft praise music playing. This was now a familiar concept, but I had a long day ahead. After a few hours, in and out of light sleep, my feet hit the floor, and I was ready to go. No more fighting. I grabbed my phone to check the time. I knew it! It was 3:00 a.m., the beginning of the fourth watch. I couldn't stay in bed; this was when miracles happened. During these precious morning hours, Jacob wrestled with God over his destiny. Moses parted the Red Sea and led the Israelites to safety and freedom. Not to mention Jesus walked on water and returned from the dead during the fourth watch. I'm not saying I ranked anywhere in the realm of these biblical giants, but I wasn't going to miss out on whatever God had in store for me. It was time for some coffee-fueled prayers.

After finishing two cups and a handful of daily devotionals, it was time to lunge into prayer. Inviting the Holy Spirit to join in and connect me to the Father was the most crucial step in profound, meaningful prayer. His presence was more tangible than I had ever experienced. A surge of electricity radiated from the top of my head and bolted down through my toes. This time he lingered like a mist rising from the water on a cool morning. He rested over me in all his peace and glory.

Wisdom fell like prophetic raindrops. Soft and gentle

yet quenching at the same time. As most spring storms build, it didn't take long for a raging storm to burst forth. Bible passages and revelations of knowledge crashed upon me. I tried my best to type them in my phone; there was no way to remember all of it. Not knowing what anything meant, my frantic fingers couldn't move fast enough. When it ended with the same abruptness as it began, I took count. Over seventy notes were captured on my phone. Were these for me? Were they topics for sermons? The words were a jumbled bowl of prophetic spaghetti, but the sun was coming out, and it was time to get to work.

When my wife left for the grocery store, I was already blazing through the yard work. There was a lengthy list ahead of me, but I was revved up and crossing things off. Her face said it all as she rounded the corner to where I was working on the front flower beds. She was in disbelief, but ecstatic the chores were getting done. "Maybe we can go out to dinner if you get done early enough," she said with a smile.

"Sounds like a plan!" I responded. Of course I'd get it done. I was on the superhighway of God's time. I could have been given ten lists, and they wouldn't have stood a chance. I had never felt so energized and full of life.

While in the groove, I checked one item off the list after another. I thought the morning couldn't get any better, but there they were. The two massive creatures my neighbors called dogs made it to their front yard. They always ignored me except for an occasional bark from time to time. The lazy kind of barking dogs do when they're old and tired. This time though, they were fixated on my every move, like wild beasts stalking prey.

Even though they were a hundred yards away, the air thickened around me. The hair on the back of my neck stood on end as adrenaline pumped through my veins. The rush of fight or flight burst on the scene, and flight wasn't on the agenda. They paced side to side, mocking me. Waiting for the command to strike.

"Here I am," I said in my spirit. "Come and get me."

Their invisible chains broke loose, and they launched into a sprint. Twenty yards and closing, fifteen, ten. "STOP!" I yelled. "You have no power here!"

The scream bellowed from deep in my spirit, but no audible words came out. Frozen in their tracks a few steps away, with teeth exposed, their snarling eased to a low rumbling growl. Commanding them to go home from within my mind, I watched as their trance faded. Life returned to their cold black eyes, and they trotted off like a couple of scolded children toward home. With all the new power coursing through my veins, I wasn't surprised. The demon dogs never stood a chance. I was now learning to walk the fragile line between natural and spiritual authority.

With all the excitement, I decided to take things one step further. It was time to test the waters, literally. How far could I push these new gifts? Peering into the clear blue water of our new swimming pool, I hung my toes off the edge of the deep end and raised both hands toward the sky in prayer. Jesus once said those who believed in him could do as he did and more. I was going to test the theory out, but after thinking it through, I figured it was better to practice over the shallow tanning ledge. Even Jesus walked from the beach before he made his way to the deep.

Resituated, it was time to focus. I extended my foot and lowered it to the crisp water. It plunged to the bottom. Nothing wrong with a practice round. I stepped back out of the water and took a deep breath. With arms outstretched like an acrobat, my foot crashed to the bottom again. Why was this not working? What did I do wrong? Maybe it was my lack of faith for not starting in the deep end. So much for being dialed in. I hunched over, sulking with my head in my hands, staring at the water.

Millions of ripples rolled across the top of the water hypnotically. My eyes tried to keep up with the fast-moving patterns as the questions for God poured out. *How do I get to where You need me? What am I missing? I know I sound like a child right now.* Frustration turned to conviction. "Lord, if You're listening, when I place the palm of my hand on the water's surface, will You make it stand still? Through You, anything is possible. Will You please do this one thing for me as a sign?"

I lowered my palm to the water as if it may never give it back. My hand rested on the surface, and I peeked through clenched eyelids. I couldn't believe it. The entire top of the pool was a sheet of glass. My own personal miracle. The ripples returned the same as before when my trembling hand was removed. The water paused for a few seconds, and they were now mine forever.

With the list whittled away to almost nothing and

with feet numb from the frigid water, it was the perfect time to clock out before the boss got home. Stepping back out of the water, it was hard to believe how blessed we were. The thought of owning a house on two acres never crossed our minds, let alone a pool to enjoy the view from. Colorful birds lined the trees and sang most days while the squirrels ran around playing grade-school tag.

Watching the pool being built was an interesting blend of excitement and frustration. The last piece of frustration had yet to be taken care of. I still had to find someone to remove concrete overspray from all the windows on the back of the house. Hazy to look through and sandpaper to the touch, they were the last remnants of construction. There was a window guy some friends used for the same thing, but he still hadn't called me back. The windows could wait, but getting ready for a rare date with the wife could not.

***

The night was supposed to be about us. After all, husband and wife relationships are the deepest connection this side of heaven. Most good dates can be defined by the level of connection, usually through conversation. The thing about meaningful conversations, though, is they typically involve more than one person speaking. I missed the memo by a mile, and she didn't get a word in on the way to the restaurant. Her relief came with the sound of my ringing cell phone. "See, honey, all in God's perfect timing," I said with a wide smile. It was the window guy calling back to schedule the cleaning.

With a sigh, she grabbed the door handle. "Can we go inside now?" she asked, already halfway out of the truck.

It was a typical Saturday at our favorite restaurant. The parking lot was lined with an array of sparkling cars and trucks, which meant we were about to have a wait ahead of us. The packed benches by the door and children kicking rocks in the landscaping pointed to a long one. We were prepared for the worst but walked unobstructed to the host stand and were taken straight to a table. Somewhere between the foyer and the table, reality faded into the background. The laughter and chatter from the tables around us dissolved into the white noise of a wind tunnel. Each step closer to the table intensified as the walls melted around us. Soon everything and everyone fell out of focus except my wife and the table. I was now seeing the world through a rain-battered window of blurred colors and blobs of movement.

Not wanting to bring attention to the altered reality around us, small talk was the best route. It didn't appear my wife could see what was happening around us as a smiling young lady walked through the blurred backdrop surrounding our table. Was she our server? As she got closer, the smile and the glow in her eyes gave it away: She was one of God's chosen people as well. How else would she have passed through to this side?

At the time, I thought God's divine intervention was giving us a perfect date amid an evil attack from the enemy. The vivid rainbow-colored walls swirling around us were beautiful and made perfect sense in the moment.

CHAPTER 2

The following week was a breeze. No battles to fight or wars to wage. This tranquility expanded my reality, one subtle layer at a time. The first came beautifully out of nowhere when the dull office transformed into a colorful painter's pallet. Bright yellow, blue, and red hues spun into hypnotic hazes atop my coworker's heads like brilliant dancing crowns. They flickered around the room, each with its own color. Try as I might, I couldn't discern their meanings, so I enjoyed the show unabridged.

At my desk, I prayed for God to grant me the eyes to see deeper and the wisdom to discern even more. My prayer was cut short by a playful, familiar voice from one of our contract drivers: a happy-go-lucky guy who bore a striking resemblance to a walking, talking ninja turtle.

From the smile protruding from his chubby face to the slight waddle as he walked through our office, the likeness was uncanny. Catching me in prayer struck up a conversation about faith and God. I'd known him for a while but had no idea his faith was so strong. As our talk continued, his physical body faded in and out, like adjusting the brightness on a computer screen. His dimmed physical body was struggling with another form, trying to explode to the surface. After a few short rounds of this, his spirit burst forth. His physical body and spiritual being were intertwined with my reality so tangibly it was hard not to reach for him.

I always knew God had a sense of humor. His spirit was the happiest creation my mind had ever fathomed, in cartoon form. It was pure joy, with no trace of pain or hardship. Untouched by our cruel and fallen world, his spirit was innocent and pure. Words will never grasp the full depth of glory his physical form gave way to. As our conversation ended and he waddled off, his spirit followed him like a balloon tied to his belt. Before turning the corner, he paused, glanced back, and winked. I questioned if he knew what I could see, and I wondered if he could see my spirit as well. There was so much to take in and so little time to figure out what it all meant.

***

The next morning rolled around, but the joy was missing. Sorrow filled my spirit to the point of drowning as fatigue laid its heavy hand on my body. Where did this come from? All week was fine, even better than usual, to be honest. The morning ride to work dragged on forever, and I debated whether to go home or continue with this miserable morning all the way to work.

Hiding my sad, out-of-character mood was as easy as hiding donuts in the break room. I'd never been good at putting on an act. Settling in at my gray corner desk, I was surrounded by bare cubicle walls in a workspace as narrow as my view of the world.

"You ready for Easter?" a voice carried over the thin dividing wall. It was Easter weekend, of course, and today was Good Friday.

"I'm not, but the kids can't wait." The words fell out of my mouth with a resounding thud as the words slide out and hit the desk. No wonder so much weight and sorrow were pressing down on me. Instead of rejoicing, I was mourning our Savior. Never had the thought crossed my mind of what Good Friday truly meant, let alone physically feeling the pain and suffering. How had I been so blind? I knew Easter would be a celebration, so I had to pull myself together. After all, not only was Easter this Sunday, but Monday was my turn to lead the work prayer meeting.

How God speaks to each of us would be my topic of discussion. Not only was I going to challenge the group to seek God's voice, I was going to unveil how God had been speaking to me during the preceding months. I wasn't sure they would believe me, but I hoped it would at least stretch their faith. God had been leaving little prophetic nuggets along the pathway of my life. I'd been doing my best to collect them as the days passed. I learned along the way how some should be picked up and kept, how some should be picked up and given to others, and how some should be put down because they weren't meant to be carried. The path, however, had evolved into a speeding train, and the prophetic nuggets were bugs smashing against the windshield. The intensity had built with each passing day, with more dots to connect and more codes to decipher.

Easter Sunday dawned with the usual fourth-watch wake-up call. The special day when death and the grave were conquered. The following five hours were filled with praise and worship music. When the rest of the house came to life, my feet were already tired from dancing. Bloodshot eyes from crying were the only remnants of an emotional whirlwind ripping through our house.

Easter service at our church had always been good, but I felt this one would be the best yet. Weaving through the crowded parking lot and squeezing through the lobby doors was like fighting an amusement park crowd. The first person we ran into was the retired pastor who had baptized not only me but my wife and daughter also. As we exchanged pleasantries, a white flame sparked above his head. It was much like the ones from work, except this color was a magnificent glow of a higher level. The rhythmic wave rising like a crown of glory was accompanied by the sound of a raging torch with echoing flames. At this point, I deduced white must be the crown of God's mighty warriors. All the words I wanted to speak about how God was moving in my life drifted beyond reach. I was in awe. After a short, one-sided conversation, we said our goodbyes and went toward the sanctuary.

Expecting a large turnout, the church had put up velvet ropes to funnel everyone into a single-file line. At first glance, this wouldn't catch anyone's eye, but an elder or two of the church stood at each open door. I had thought it was crowd control the year prior, but a higher purpose became clear as we inched our way to the front. The same glow enshrouding our old pastor's head moments earlier also radiated from each of the elders. They were the gatekeepers of the church. Most people, including the hired security guards, saw through worldly eyes. These men, however, were the true watchmen for the church. I had no doubt they saw through the veil as their authority burst forth into the natural realm. I almost couldn't bring myself to shake the elder's hand as we reached the doors, but passing up the opportunity wasn't an option.

The Easter service was fantastic, and the rest of the day was a blur.

The following day was my Monday to lead the prayer meeting, and the anticipation had been driving me nuts. I knew the little prophetic nuggets I had collected over the weeks prior would blow their minds. This would be life-changing for all of us. I was bouncing through the office when one of our company founders strolled by. I couldn't pass it up. He had to join us. I threw out the invitation, and he must have sensed the excitement in my voice, because he agreed to sit in with us. Nine-thirty couldn't come fast enough.

I took my usual seat at the table earlier than usual. The industrial room, with light-painted block walls, was more alive and beautiful than ever. On the two longer sides were a decorative mirror and a vibrant print of a bluebonnet field. Below them stood two faux-wood hutches running half the room's length. Even the stone tabletop, with its sprawling grains like a majestic oak, drew my attention like never before. On the left wall hung a whiteboard and to the right was a television. It was there, on the television, where I would show them the incredible way God spoke to me. With my back to the bluebonnets and my hands tracing the flowing grains, I knew things were about to change. Neither I, nor my wife, were prepared for how right I was about to be.

The next hour would be a thrill ride with an arsenal of church-service clips, Bible verses, and firsthand experiences. I went through my phone and opened many tabs, so they were ready to project on the television. There was too much to fit into this one-hour meeting, but I had to try. If they knew all of it, they might think I was a little crazy anyway.

The room filled right on time, but it was a shame no more than six people could sit at the table. I wanted everyone to see what was about to happen. The next twenty minutes played out like a dream. Mania took over, but, much like a train, if you've never seen one before, the vibrating tracks below your feet meant nothing. I jumped from this video to that experience, back to a string of numbers connecting like a secret code. My presentation finished with a Christian music video containing a hidden meaning only I seemed to understand. It flew by like someone had smashed the fast-forward button, and everyone was along for the ride. Before anyone spoke, I revealed "The Way." The Way was the name of the church we had to build, and God had called me to pastor.

"Did you catch everything wrapped in the coded numbers and video collage?" I asked. "This is the second time God has called me to be a pastor. This time I'm saying,

'Here I am, God, send me.'"

They looked around at each other, speechless. Of course they were silent. I would be, too, if I were them.

"We're supposed to build the biggest church ever, a present-day Noah's ark. How cool would it be to build a modern-day ark?" I asked them, jumping to my feet.

A small discussion followed, but nothing too deep. They didn't see it as I did. After all, it was meant for me and not for them. God had shown me the future, and He would show it to them so they could understand, when the time was right. I had no doubt construction plans would be drawn up on our new state-of-the-art megachurch shortly after. They needed to get the ball rolling sooner than later, though. We had so little time to save millions of people before the rapture. I was about to have a lot of work to do myself. After all, I still hadn't figured out how to fit seminary in around work. Maybe they would send me there instead of reporting to work. But, then again, did I need to be taught anything? My relationship with God was so close I was sure He would show me everything. It was God's plan, though, so I wasn't going to waste time worrying.

If nothing else, I wanted to be included in the church design. After all, the blueprints had been given to me in a vision. The main church would sit on forty-five acres of land our company owned thirty minutes north of our central office. The administration offices would rest on the fifteen acres they owned down the road from the forty-five.

I saw the road map clear as day, step by step. At the time, there wasn't a rail line on the property. The first step would be constructing one to run through the back side of the land. The rail would have a three-fold purpose in creating The Way. First, it would be the fastest way to move massive amounts of building materials to the construction site. The second purpose was to be fulfilled after construction was complete. We would transform it into a rail system for transporting people so they could be saved by the thousands. The final, most crucial phase of the rail system would come to pass for our children's children. Their generation would need an ark like Noah's. The Way would be a haven for God's chosen children. The rail would be the lifeline for transporting people, food, and the supplies needed to survive.

I knew an economic downturn would happen. As a

company in the construction industry, we would be able to keep so many good people in business as we built this sanctuary. The rest of the world would struggle to keep their head above water, but God would supply more blessings for and through us than anyone could fathom. The work would take many years and involve thousands of workers and millions of dollars. We would choose the right companies to partner with, and God would do the heavy lifting for us.

When everyone thinks of the end times, they think of doom, wrath, pain, and starvation. God showed me how we are His children and how He would carry us through any fire, the same as we protect our own children. As the Bible says, all the terrible events leading to the end of times would happen, and we were to be the beacon of hope for the lost. God would unite the many godly companies during this time to stand firm and provide for His kingdom. Each was a valuable member of the same body, and there would be abundant food, fuel, water, and joy during those times, as long as we built a refuge.

Our refuge would be The Way, and we would build it. The main building for the church would come first after the installation of the rail line. Shaped like a massive stadium from the outside, it would put all other structures to shame. This was supposed to be the first church where every person would be paid for their time and effort. From full-time staff to part-time help, God wanted us to care for His people. Paying for it would be simple by bringing in famous Christian bands from all over the country who would sell out shows. Concerts Friday and Saturday, followed by Sunday morning praise to kick off the service. The bands would make money for their time, and the church would make money to keep the lights on. This setup would bring people through the doors who might never attend otherwise.

After a few years of momentum, it would be time to construct the perimeter walls. Building the massive walls around the forty-five acres would take years. Like Jerusalem's walls, they had to be strong enough to withstand the enemy's attack during the end times and be built piece by piece at God's command. The entry gates would be the last and most ornate pieces constructed on the property. This critical piece would be left to our grandchildren to design. We couldn't blow our cover right from the start. God wanted us to build and strengthen His people and His complex without catching the watchful eye of the enemy.

The rest of the week was spent clawing through the repetitive motions of work with my head down. The founder had told me I had better start by preaching to people around the office, but my coworkers seemed to vanish. The office seemed rather quiet, and I wondered if they took me seriously. Were they working on the plan behind the scenes, and I was out of the loop? Maybe they were getting paperwork in order and funding together. I was sure they would bring me into the loop when it was time to break ground. I had to bide my time studying the Word and getting closer to His presence.

The first step was to get my son baptized to protect him under God's grace like the rest of our family. The day finally arrived for him to take the next step of faith and get baptized. It was the day we broke generational curses for good. I hadn't failed as a father. I had helped bring him to the best decision he could ever make.

We didn't sit in our usual seats at church, which are usually in the back rows. Instead, we sat a few rows from the baptistry at the front. I was overflowing with excitement and joy. My wife had a firm grip on my hand as though I was tethered to her. I would have floated to the ceiling if she hadn't held on. The praise music began, and the doors opened. The line moved in, and my little buddy was in the middle. His excitement choked out his shyness, and the crowd didn't bother him.

"Would you like to help baptize your son?" asked one of our friends overseeing the line. Before my wife could clench my hand harder, I was already in on the action. Before I knew it, my son climbed the steps to the basin and plunged into the water. The pastor said a few words, and we leaned him back in unison. Bursting forth through the water came a brand-new child of God. One with eternal life in the kingdom of God. It was a beautiful moment. My whole family was protected for eternity; the physical world could never harm them.

Afterward, we walked hand in hand down the hallway toward the bathroom so he could change. "My legs were shaking so bad," he said, looking up at me.

"It took a lot of courage to stand up in front of all those people, buddy," I said as we rounded the corner to the bathrooms.

"Does that mean I'm brave, Dad?"

"That's exactly what it means, buddy."

When the service ended, they had a table set up for the people who had been baptized. Lots of cool things lined the table, including Bibles for all ages. After combing through the items, my son grabbed a colorful children's Bible, and we bounced toward the doors.

We were a few feet from the front door when the executive pastor caught my eye. "You and the kids go to the truck, honey; I'll catch up in a minute," I told my wife, tossing her the keys like they were on fire. Earlier, during service, the executive pastor had passed the lead role to his successor: a younger man, full of faith and fire. I had never spoken to either of them before, but I was on a mission to tell them how excited I was.

"Hey, pastor, any chance I can speak to you and our new lead pastor for a minute?" I asked.

"Sure thing, wait right here," he said. "Don't go anywhere."

He disappeared into the crowd, and a familiar face slid between me and the sea of people filling the lobby. The young man before me sang with the worship team most Sundays. Small in stature, he wore a suit jacket big enough to fit him and a few friends combined. He stared joyfully at me and asked, "How have you been lately? You seem so happy."

As he spoke, the world slowed to a crawl. His eyes glazed over and bulged into large, polished marbles. I wondered if this was an angel or a demon.

"I've been doing great, and so has the family," I said, attempting to discern if it was an honest question or the first move in an evil chess game. "Trying to live every day for Jesus. How about you?" I thought the question would shake it out of him one way or another.

"Absolutely!" he said, unable to fold his eyelids over the massive, cartoonish objects he now had for eyes. With a swooping, ear-to-ear smile, he left to mingle with passersby. It was an angel. With complete certainty, an angel must have taken over his body. Unless he had always been an angel in disguise.

I was still wired from my encounter when both pastors emerged from the crowd and stood before me. I couldn't believe these two mighty men of God were right here in front of me. What happened next was nothing short of a catapult launch. All the thoughtful and encouraging things I wanted to speak about were ransacked by random thoughts spewing like a busted fire hose. A few minutes in, they politely interrupted and asked me to email them about the rest. This was a relief for me and, judging by their faces, for them as well. I wasn't sure what happened, but I knew I could sit down and draft an email without nerves taking over. All the excitement was getting to me.

As evening settled in and the excitement calmed, it was Bible and prayer time with my son. He had a daily devotional and a Bible we read each night before bed. I noticed he still had the toy he had gotten from Sunday school in his hand. It looked like one of those Chinese finger traps from when I was a child, except both ends were sewn shut, and it had a single black marble in it. There was also a pattern of three diamonds on it. The three diamonds stood for the Holy Trinity, but I wondered what the single marble stood for. It only made sense it stood for the chosen one, but who was chosen for what? Was he the chosen one, or was he meant to give it to me as a sign? What if he was chosen, and we were building The Way for him to preach at? After reading and prayer, I asked if he would let me take the toy to work, and he reluctantly agreed. He pointed to his new Bible from church on his desk and asked if we could read it when we finished the old one. Before leaving his room, I flipped through the pages. "This Bible needs to go back to the church. It has too much confusion in it. Too many pictures, games, and puzzles. God's Word shouldn't be diluted like this," I said as I snapped the Bible shut and smacked it on the desk.

The evening ended, and I was still filled with energy to the point that an audible humming noise should have emanated from my body. Each night had been more diffi-cult to fall asleep than the previous, with restless minutes turning into hours. I was tumbling in bed like a rock in a dryer.

At some point, I grabbed my wife's hand for comfort, and my fingers met a chilling terror. She was ice-cold, like there was no life in her body. Touching her clammy face, she flinched as my hand grazed her skin. She was still alive, but for how much longer? I put my face within inches of hers and began praying. Fear gripped my entire being as adrenaline shot through my veins. Death had entered our room, and he was trying to take her from me. A black mass, darker than the moonless night, towered over the foot of the bed. I held her in my arms and prayed with fury to keep him at arm's length.

Death, however, waltzed around the room, taunting, and waiting for a chance to strike. I couldn't bring myself to confront him for fear he'd snatch us both. Chills ripped through my body like razors as the sound of his robe drug the floor and consumed the room like a funeral march. "Jesus defeated death and the grave; you have no power here," I whispered with a wishful, but quivering voice. Two could play this game. Standing guard all night in prayer over my wife while he paced the room was easy enough, considering the adrenaline and my usual lack of sleep. At the sound of her alarm, she rolled over to turn it off, and I whispered, "We made it, honey. We made it."

CHAPTER 3

All day at work, I could only think about getting home. How was Death himself able to stroll right into our home? There had to be an entry point for evil spirits to slither their way in, and I wondered what it could be. We wrote Bible verses on all the framed entryways when our home was built. We had always prayed at the dinner table and at bedtime. Our house should have been an impenetrable fortress. I wasn't sure what to look for when I got home, but five o'clock couldn't come soon enough.

Halfway home, the blinders gave way to revelation. It had to be the patinaed metal sign hanging in the garage a lifelong friend had given me. He carved my last name with care and craft from a solid metal sheet for my last birthday. What I forgot to consider when he gave it to me was the fact that his house had been haunted a few months prior. Malevolent spirits had harassed him and his family. They caught crazy things on camera that would make an average person's skin crawl. Not my buddy, though. He fought it head-on with the help of multiple pastors and God on his side. Undoubtedly, he had given me more than a sign for my birthday.

When I arrived home, I realized this was not the sole dent in our armor. An old burn barrel at the back of our property had to be the other. I had burnt precious pieces of God's creation without remorse on a rusty altar. How could I have done such a thing and not been aware? I should be ashamed for having reduced God's glorious creations to nothing but coals and ash.

I tore into the driveway on a mission, and the fence behind the drive almost became the first opponent. It took willpower not to break into a full-on sprint. The heavy steel gate at the back of the yard squealed as it flew open. The noise could have drawn attention, but it was better than leaping or falling over the fence at my age. This part of the yard led to a circular opening down by a winding creek, outlined by towering trees as old as they were tall.

I slowed to a walk as I reached the center. The decrepit altar sat on its pedestal, mocking my every step. I ripped it from the cinder block base with a sharp grunt and hurled it toward the tree line. *Good riddance,* I thought as I puffed my chest out in victory.

Making my way up the hill and around the truck, I dropped the tailgate with a thud. Out of breath, I went inside the garage. There it was, hanging on the wall, the catalyst for the intense standoff the night before. The possessed sign had lain dormant for months, but it was time to show the enemy who was boss. I ripped it from the wall and slammed it in the truck.

As the tailgate slammed shut in victory, I paused for a moment of silence, looking around. A small metal cannon living on a corner shelf caught my eye. The brass barrel and stainless-steel frame had lost their shine long ago. The barrel was bored out and had a small hole at the back where a wick would go if it were life-sized. It had been a small part of me since I was young. Pretend as I might, it still meant something. I had managed not to lose it after all these years. My father made the cannon in a metal shop class. As a child, I would sometimes pretend he made it for me. My need for his affection faded long ago, leaving only a few tattered memories.

I never had the chance to love my father, and this trinket was the sole tangible thing I remember receiving from him. The shock on his face when my grandmother and I pulled up to his shop class will forever be ingrained in my memory. After the short burst of surprise on his face wore off, he climbed into the car and handed me this miniature cannon in the back seat. At the time, I couldn't believe he was handing it over. The weight in my hand was great for something so small in stature. Each part moved like a real cannon, even the squeaky wheels. Not five minutes into playing, the barrel smacked the frame like a mousetrap and snared my finger. I held back tears with everything I had so he wouldn't take it back. To my surprise, he never did; I've had it ever since.

He passed away a couple of years ago, and this was all I had to show for his life, a toy never intended for me in the first place. How much bad energy had clung to it over the years? It moved with me from state to state and house to house, but now seemed like the time to let it go. I felt its weight one last time on the way to the truck. I said one last farewell while the tailgate lowered, and it slipped through my fingers like the fading memory of what could have been.

Falling to the truck bed, it slammed like a half-read book shutting forever. The horn blared and sent me flying through the air with the closing of the tailgate. The radio screamed and the dashboard exploded into a light show. Shouting, "Not today!" I ran for the cab of the truck. Almost ripping the door from the hinges, I smashed the ignition on the dash. After several brutal seconds, the lights and sounds subsided. "I told you I wasn't playing. You're not welcome here," I screamed. The neighbors would have thought I was crazy if they had been outside, but I was too livid to care.

Laying down this level of spiritual authority with force was becoming second nature. The bursts of hallucinations were sliding in seamlessly with greater intensity and coming more often. I couldn't believe how long it took to peel the scales from my blind eyes. *A gift and a curse,* I thought, but I wouldn't have changed it for the world.

The house should be clear, but I was no stranger to the twilight hours and planned to stand guard. Lack of sleep, I

JAMES COAST

would find out weeks later, was one of the most significant signs of mania when accompanied by zero signs of fatigue. In my case, I felt better and more alive than ever.

Another sleepless night gave way to beeping alarm clocks. Not a single unexpected noise was heard, and, best of all, no uninvited guests crashed my party. I was full of energy and buzzing like a fluorescent lightbulb. Running on what I thought was God's time felt amazing.

Halfway through the morning, my phone chirped, and a text message sparked my memory. It was the lead purchasing agent from one of our largest customers. We were supposed to meet for lunch, and I had flat-out forgotten. Thank goodness he reached out. It would have been unprofessional of me not to show up. Pulling the phone close, the text said: *Let's meet at the steakhouse at I-35 and Pleasant Run Rd between noon and one*. What kind of weird code was this? Not only did he not give an exact time, but he also didn't give an exact place. Was it possible my phone was tapped, so he was being intentionally vague? Was he on my side and didn't want us to be followed, or was it a setup?

Let's do twelve-thirty on the dot, I sent back, suspicious of who else might be reading the messages. If he responded with a straight answer, it would surely be safe for lunch. The chirp of a thumbs-up emoji interrupted what was now weaving into a full-blown conspiracy theory. He was smart. How was I supposed to decode a cartoon hand? Set up or not, I no longer feared anything in this world. With a few exciting encounters under my belt already, a simple lunch would be an easy enough adventure. The cross streets were about an hour away, add an hour for lunch, plus the drive back. I had enough time to let my coworkers know I'd be gone for a while before hitting the road.

I pushed through the front doors as I had a thousand times before and caught a glimpse of the makeshift sign hanging on the stone wall. It had been placed when Covid gripped the nation. The faded wooden rectangle leaning to one side was the last remnant of the pandemic of fear. The worn surface made it hard to see the outlined picture of a person's face being swallowed by a mask. It was time for this sign to find a new home, and I knew where it belonged. It popped from the wall with a yank, leaving one crooked little nail behind.

I unlocked the truck from ten feet away as the neighbor a few feet beyond the tailgate came into view. A single-wide trailer with old cars in the front and clutter in the back rested on the property next door. The enemy had set up shop there long ago and had been watching us. The old me would have been scared and frozen, but not anymore.

Staring at the neighbor as I rounded the truck toward the tailgate, I realized he hadn't raised his head once. Shovel in hand, he was working feverishly to dig a hole. Any normal person digging in their yard wouldn't be suspicious. They would be planting a tree or bush, perhaps flowers. However, this one wore solid black dress clothes from top to bottom and dug without progress. Not a single scoop of dirt had come out yet. In fact, the man was wrestling the shovel out of the shallow hole like it was stuck in a tar pit. His motions repeated, a five-second loop of revolving frustration. It was evident God had entangled him so I could make the lunch meeting without delay. A few feet from the man in black, the wood sign found its new home next to the metal one. The tailgate slammed, and I cut my eyes toward the gravedigger, but nothing. He didn't flinch.

Behind the wheel, I paused to reflect, and another

person caught my eye, mid-parking lot. *Leave*, I told myself, looking at the exit. *I can't be late.* The man shuffling about in the middle of the parking lot got the better of me, though. He was pacing in front of the stone walls by the gate leading to the loading area. He couldn't get past the snarling lion heads standing guard. What a sight it was to see them in action.

Ten feet left, ten feet right, pause. Ten feet left, ten feet right, pause. He paced back and forth but made no forward movement. With world-conquering confidence, I walked up behind him. He spun around, eyes wide, when I tapped his shoulder, and his quickness caused me to stumble. The whites of his eyes were polished cue balls stamped dead center with bottomless black diamond pupils. I told myself he was a person, nothing more than a fellow human being. The enemy takes possession of non-believers as he chooses, hopping from one to the next.

"Can I help you, sir?" I asked between air-stealing heartbeats. No answer, but he glared straight through me, raising his receipt. It looked legit. Something must have taken control when he was trying to get loaded. Maybe the neighbor had something to do with this, but he was gone. No shovel, no neighbor. Back to the vessel in front of me. He returned his arm to his side, receipt in hand. Our eyes met again, and my reflection appeared in a pair of normal brown eyes.

"I'll call someone to load you, sir," I said. "Hang tight." I couldn't figure out if multiple spirits were trying to rattle me or if one was jumping from body to body to distract me.

Back in front of the steering wheel, uncertainty hit. What was this lunch for again? Did he know about my new abilities? We had attempted to go to lunch for weeks, but they kept getting canceled. The questions spun over and over while I left the parking lot. The signs in my truck bed, of course. If he asked for a sign, it was a setup. It meant he wanted to confirm I had found my unique gifting before throwing me in his trunk. I made a plan, though. I would drop the tailgate and tell him I had two, one metal, one wood, and he could take his pick. It should throw him off the scent enough to buy a little time. Everything happens for a reason, and those signs might be helpful.

Driving, I scrolled through the map and almost got close enough to drop a pin, when the phone rang, obscuring the screen. Decline, dang it. Finding the cross streets again, the same number stole the screen a second time. Giving up, I tossed the phone aside. Besides, wherever I ended up was where I was supposed to be.

Heading south down the freeway, the radio shorted out. Flashing on, then going silent over and over. Turning the unit on and off a few times didn't help. This wasn't a coincidence; it had to be bugged. Someone—or worse, something—was tracking me. I jabbed at the touchscreen buttons, blurting out, "I know you're listening." The screen turned black mid-sentence, then shot back on at ear-piercing decibels. Fighting back, I finally turned it off, opting for silence.

Cruising in silence heightened my senses. A brilliant cherry-red semi passed on the left. I had never seen such a rich and beautiful color. Many more spectacular colors followed. A small, still voice spoke out between the roar of cars and passing trucks: *Tall glass of water.* What did that mean? I knew it was God, but I didn't understand. Merging right, I took the exit toward where the lunch was supposed to take place. *A tall glass of water.* I would find out at some point what that meant.

The off-ramp led up a gradual incline, and the steak-house was on the right, tucked away off the busy freeway. I had to be able to grab a sign if prompted, so I pulled forward into a parking space with fear piercing through my concentration. What if my phone and truck had been tapped for months, and I was playing right into their game? Who were they, and what did they want from me? Conspiracy theories were never my thing, but anxiety was sinking its hooks in little by little.

The loose stainless-steel watch dangling from my wrist confirmed I had arrived early. It, along with my baggy clothes, also confirmed I was losing weight at a rapid pace, but neither myself nor anyone else had caught on. I hid my phone in the console, and it landed on my son's small marble toy from church. I forgot it was in there, tucked away nice and neat, like a prize jewel. I stuffed it in my pocket in case they were after it.

The sun was shining, and I didn't want to let it go to waste. I didn't often enjoy the cool breeze and singing birds during the workweek. The air filled with the wafting scent of mesquite wood billowing from the rooftop behind me as the truck door swung open. *What a beautiful day it is turning out to be,* I thought as my feet hit the ground and the door slammed behind me. I'd never been to lunch on this side of town. Twirling the marble toy in my pocket, I stepped over the curb onto a grassy area. Was this the beginning of the rest of my life, or was this how it all ended? Would I be kidnapped and thrown in a trunk, or was I here to meet the guide for my new gifting? Could this be a regular lunch I was thinking way too much into? No, this was anything but ordinary. I felt it in my soul.

The internal debate was halted as my eyes caught two poles a few feet off the parking lot. The first was a weathered wooden pole splintered with age. Some of the purest materials on the planet were wooden objects like this. Made from trees and nothing else, so simple, yet so beautiful. Man has been building life-altering things since the dawn of time out of plain and simple wood. The second pole was metal. Much taller than the first, this was a square tube crying blood-stained tears of rust. It was rotting away in sadness, much like society.

Movement in the distance broke through my curious observations about the poles. A hundred yards away and down a hill appeared to be another business. Trying to determine what it was led me further away from the parking lot. No visible signs or markings, my curiosity drew me in. The sweet smell of juicy steaks and mesquite wood faded with each step. At first, the new odor was weak and unrecognizable, but it didn't take long to overtake me. My eyes began to water as the stench of sulfur snaked its gnarled fingers around my throat and attempted to steal the life from my lungs. Frozen, unable to gasp, the evil was tangible.

The beautiful spring day I had left behind moments ago was beyond my grasp. Evil was coming from the building. It looked like pure death down the hill surrounding the cabin-like building. The landscape was obscured and oppressive, with dried grass and barren trees. The sun itself was scared to shine upon it. Grasping for each breath, through a teary-eyed gaze, I watched as a lady appeared in the doorway. Too far to make out words, her body language said it all. She was on a frantic call flailing about as if someone had died. The place was ripe with anxiety and soul-stealing trauma. It wasn't my battle, though; I had other plans. I wasn't strong enough to take on whatever lurked inside those walls. Heart pounding in my chest, I made a break for fresh air.

Turning uphill toward the truck, I took a few steps forward and felt the air already lighter. Now able to breathe, I glanced down the hill one last time, but the lady was gone. Only terror remained, seeping through the walls. Between us was an odd formation of trees. I was so focused I must have walked right by them. Two massive trees were joined in the shape of a towering arch. The tree on the left was full of vibrant green leaves, like the tree of life leaning in for a kiss. On the right, a lifeless and barren tree of death had latched to the living one. This was no kiss; it was a battle of life and death. The slight breeze accentuated the deadly dance as each side struggled to gain ground. It wasn't an ordinary archway formed by accident. It was a portal of death, which now explained the stench and building behind it. I stood in wonder. How many people had died by walking under the archway, disappearing forever? Or worse yet, did vile things from another realm use it to come through to this side?

This was too much to fathom on an empty stomach. It was twelve-thirty on the dot. Time to head back to the restaurant, where more cars had filled the parking lot.

Good, now there were plenty of witnesses in case something crazy happened. As my feet hit the pavement, a disturbing pattern of blacked-out cars and SUVs unfolded. Some had engines still rumbling, and all stood between me and the door. The familiar heartbeat sound built to a steady thump between my ears, pounding with every step toward destiny. If they wanted me, they had a fight on their hands. I trusted that whatever was about to happen was supposed to happen, but it didn't mean I couldn't take a few swings. I walked up the sidewalk past them, head down, concentrating on my feet. It appeared like I would enjoy lunch after all as I passed them unobstructed and turned the corner.

CHAPTER 4

The sweet aroma of baked bread and hand-cut steaks replaced the remaining trace of sulfur as the solid wood doors gave way to the foyer. A little old lady with wrinkled slacks and a half-tucked-in shirt scurried by as menus slipped through her fingertips, saying, "I'll be right with you, sir."

The dining area was void of sunlight. Aside from a few shadowy outlines scattered among the tables, it was difficult to see how empty the place was. The hostess ran around frantically, but only one group needed to be sat, and she blew right by them without looking up. Not sure I blamed her; the mix of long trench coats and business attire made them hard to read. A tense conversation in a foreign tongue arose from the middle of the group, but it didn't offer any insight. They could have been busi-nessmen, cops, or perhaps a hired hit squad. *Maybe they would be polite enough to let me enjoy my last meal if they were hitmen.* As I finished my thought, the straggler of the group shot me a look as if I had yelled in his face. Was he able to hear my thoughts? With a smirk, his attention returned to the group as the hostess reappeared to usher them to the dining area.

I had been so caught up trying to figure those guys out, two more had snuck in behind me. Clean cut, mid-thirties at best, these two were my kind of company. One may have been who I was there to meet and brought a coworker.

"It sure is nice out there today. What brings you two in today, besides lunch, of course?" My question broke through their casual conversation.

Without missing a beat, they turned in my direction. "We're passing through on business," the taller one replied, putting his hands in his pockets.

"You two wouldn't happen to be meeting someone here for lunch, would you? I'm waiting on a client I've never met in person."

"Nope, just us taking a break from the grind," said the

second gentleman.

Still not who I was here to meet. "Well, you guys enjoy your lunch and have a great afternoon," I said, turning my attention to the stressed, little gray-haired hostess.

"Are you three dining together?" she asked, reaching for the stack of menus.

"No, but I'm expecting someone else, so I'll need a table for two, please."

Nodding, she grabbed two menus and motioned for me to follow her straight ahead to the bar area. My heart grew heavy as I followed her, when I realized work for her wasn't a choice. I couldn't imagine what a busy day did to the poor old lady. It wouldn't be long before she had a heart attack at the rate she was going.

"Here you go," she said, stopping at a booth and laying the menus down. "You can sit facing the door to see when your guest arrives."

As she walked off, something didn't add up. Why did she want me to face the door? Her nerves were shot, and she was not even partway through the day. I couldn't trust her, so I sat on the other side of the booth with my back to the door. I wasn't worried if someone would come up behind me. "Let go and let God," is what people always say. I wasn't scared of the sketchy people lurking around or any new ones walking through the front door.

A big-screen television hung on the wall straight ahead, and a second mirrored it on the far side of the liquor shelves. The U-shaped bar was on my right, and the two guys from the foyer were sitting at the far corner of it. They seemed nice, and I was glad they were sitting close. Maybe they'd jump in and help me if something went down. The outside edge of the room was lined with booths, of which many were empty. An exit to the parking lot was cut in the wall at the room's farthest side. Not easy to get to, but I'd never been much of a runner anyway. I attempted to settle in for the ride.

The silverware clanged against the wooden table from unraveling the cloth napkin, and I was reminded of the poles outside. Metal versus wood, God's creation versus man's creation. I centered my finger on the wooden handle of the steak knife and gave it a whirl on the table. How could I not pause and admire both elements working hand in hand? The knife made with wood and metal has done so much throughout history. It has been a staple in our society for taking lives and saving them. *Life is all about balance,* spun in my head, while the knife rotated as if winding a clock backward.

Each turn of the knife ripped more air from my lungs until nothing was left. Paralyzed, all but my crooked fingers and thoughts stilled as the world slowed to a crawl around me. Panic set in as the struggle for air was lost in a silent battle. With nothing left to give, the familiar odor of death and sulfur seeped through the air and crept back into my lungs. Something was following me, something powerful. I hoped it wasn't my lunch guest walking in the door.

"Hi there. Can I get you something to drink?" the waitress asked, leaning in. Her voice floated by, echoing through the darkness of a long tunnel. "Hello, rough day at work?" she tried again.

This time it sounded close enough that I could see the way out as both my hands slammed the spinning knife to a stop.

"Water, please," I replied with a tremble that straightened her smile.

"Are you ready to order yet?" she asked, clenching

down on her notepad.

"I'm still waiting for someone. He should be here any minute," I said, forcing a smile. How could she talk in this gas chamber?

"I'll be right back," she said. Her smile returned as another guy sat behind her at the closest corner of the bar.

He isn't who I'm waiting on, or he would have sat down across from me, I thought, glancing at my watch. Twelve forty-five; some people are always late. He was either way late, or this was a ploy to get me here alone. The air was so thick I wasn't sure I would be able to eat even if he did show up. No one else was reacting to the intense rotten-egg odor escaping from the walls. Whatever it was must have been trying to scare me off, but I was there for a reason, and I wasn't leaving until I figured it out. The waitress sat my water down and greeted the new guy at the bar. Could "tall glass of water" have something to do with her or the glass in front of me? *It isn't tall,* I thought while lifting the glass to inspect for remnants of poison. Why was I questioning God anyway? If it was supposed to be poisoned, it was supposed to be poisoned. He would either keep me alive or take me home. Who was I to second-guess anything?

Maybe reading the menu would kill some time without bringing unwanted attention. The words were hard to make out because the only light came from the televisions across the bar. Both were set to the same sports channel and must have been playing the best sporting fights of all time, judging by all the black eyes and bruises. A dugout-emptying fight was followed by a bloody hockey boxing match. The violence made it hard to watch. The chaotic sports brawls led to a closeup of a man's head being stomped while he tried to cover his face. As the camera panned out, it was clear it was a mob beating or a protest ending in violence. I thought it was a sports channel, but given the atmosphere of this place, I guess it made sense at the time.

I turned my attention to the room, wondering where the waitress had gone. So caught up in the show, I hadn't noticed all the chatter from the other tables had ceased. Not only had the conversations frozen but so had the people. Not a single movement, like statues in a deserted garden at dusk. A chill slithered through my bones as my focus returned to the television. It was the same violent clips repeating. Time had frozen around me. An older fellow leaning in the side entrance was stuck on the same loop as the screens. He wore a light brown fedora and giant sunglasses, which were held in place by ears rivaling in size. He poked his head in from underneath the exit sign. Stiff old fingers clutched the doorway as he leaned in—looking left, looking right—then withdrew. Round and round he went as if trying to find someone or something.

What now, though? How was I supposed to get everyone unstuck? As a grim reality set in, I planted my face on the table like a child in timeout. What if the entire world was wrapped in this stench and stuck forever?

I was searching through the darkness for answers in the deep corners of my soul when a faint voice shattered the silence around me. "Would you like some bread while you wait?"

Bread? Who would eat bread at a time like this? I lifted my head to the familiar voice enough to peek over my crossed arms. It was the waitress, and she was animated again like nothing had happened. Jolting upright, I scanned the room. What a relief. Everyone was moving.

"Yes, that would be great," I said, remembering God prepares a table for us before our enemies. I may not be surrounded by friends, but I wouldn't pay any attention to whatever was messing with me. The old man in the doorway was already sitting at the bar, facing my direction. Speaking of enemies, was he one of them? He snuck in the side door, after all. I might have missed my chance to run while everyone was frozen.

"Here you go," the waitress said, setting down the bread and severing my train of thought.

I would eat and savor each bite, even if this bread was poisoned. My God would protect me, and I would be on the fast path to heaven even if he didn't. Whittling the bread down to nothing took forever. After all, I had to prove a point. The waitress stopped by again. "Are you ready to order? I don't think your friend is going to show up."

She was right, and I thought it best to keep the game moving forward. "I'll have whichever steak you want to bring me, medium, and whatever side you think is best."

Folding her notebook over and stuffing it in her apron, she said, "Easy enough."

As she was about to walk off, I interrupted with, "Hey, let me pay the tab for those two guys sitting at the corner of the bar. I was planning to buy someone's lunch anyway."

Nodding in agreement, she made it three whole steps away from the table before snapping back. "You're going to tip me for their lunch, too, right?" she said, squinting her eyes with a crinkled-up nose. This time it was my turn to nod in agreement as relief came to her face. She must have been struggling to make ends meet with how concerned she was over a lunch-order tip.

My steak arrived at the table, and so did my new friends. On their way to the door, the guys from the bar stopped to thank me for picking up their tab and left a business card. The small talk was short and friendly, with them in a hurry to return to work and me staring at a steak. I glanced at the card while setting it down to grab the fork. One of them owned a multifamily construction company. Maybe they had something to do with the church we would build. The card may have been the whole reason for the lunch excursion.

I signed the receipt and stuffed the business card in my wallet after stuffing my face. About to slide from the booth, a young man barely old enough to work appeared from around the bar. He was coming toward me with a metal pitcher, so I sank back into the seat. He reached the booth and raised the pitcher.

"Can I refill your water, sir?"

Here we go. This was the "tall glass of water," echoing from earlier. "Yes, thank you," I said, lifting my glass.

He tilted the pitcher and began pouring the water. His human eyes were snatched from his face and rolled back in his head. The emptiness was replaced by serpent eyes. A forked tongue lashed from his mouth as he pulled the pitcher back to his chest. Frozen for a moment, I knew what this was now.

"How are you doing today?" I asked, trying to reach the poor boy trapped inside.

"I'm freaking out. I'm leaving soon for a job interview. It's at a body shop, and I hope it's a brand-new life for me," he said as the pitcher shook. His eyes flashed between human and horror with each word as he wrestled with fear over his future.

"Can I pray for you?" I asked, reaching for his shoulder. He agreed, and as my hand rested on his bony shoulder, I prayed with power over his life and future. The enemy wasn't taking this one, not if I could help it. When

I said amen and opened my eyes, tears built in his soft human eyes as he leaned in for a hug to say thank you. "You're going to have a blessed life, kid. Keep fighting," I whispered, and walked off.

Pleased from having made it through lunch in one piece, I almost didn't notice the rogue foot sticking out from the corner on my way toward the door. Plopped back in a chair with her legs sprawled out, it appeared the little old hostess had enough of this place. As she stared toward the ceiling, she waved a menu back and forth in her small, fragile hand. I was glad she was still alive, but there was no way I was hanging around for pleasantries. A few steps from the wooden doors, I hoped they worked in reverse. They were big and heavy for a reason. What if they were made to trap me inside? I didn't have a backup plan or my phone to call for help. I held back the urge to charge the doors, but the echo of my footsteps got louder and louder, bouncing inside the walls of my head. With a desperate push, the surrounding darkness gave way to the soft embrace of the sun. It was so easy to take the sun for granted until I wasn't sure I would see it again.

The air was clean and fresh. What a shame I had to go

back to work. Wondering how long I had been trapped for lunch, I checked my watch, and it was dead. It had stopped dead on twelve forty-five, the last time I checked it. It had never given out on me before, but something had sucked the power from the battery. Now in the truck, I turned on my cell phone to check the time. The lock screen flashed one thirty-five as a stream of dings from missed text messages piled up.

In the mix of missed messages was one from my missing lunch counterpart. At twelve twenty-five, he wrote, *Are you here?* Followed by a second message at twelve fifty-five, *I didn't hear from you, so I ended up leaving.* I was standing in the doorway at twelve-thirty. There was no way I walked through the parking lot right by him as he sat there. This didn't sit right. Why wouldn't he come inside the restaurant? Formulating a response to play dumb, I wrote, *Oh, no! I must have gone to the wrong one! I just got done eating by myself. Well, not really, we never eat alone. I'm so sorry! I wondered what had happened, but I left my phone in the truck so we could eat in peace. Let me know if I can make it up to you, sir.*

I wanted to see if he could work his way around my

response. The only steakhouse in the area was the one in my rearview mirror. Five minutes later, he responded, *All good. These things happen. I was outside waiting but didn't go inside. We can always try again, buddy. Just let me know. Buddy? How dare he call me buddy; that's my word. Who schedules lunch but doesn't get out of their car?* It made no sense to me.

With so much to process, my mind reeled with excitement and theories. They were churning so fast it was hard to grasp any as they melted together and burned off before any solid ideas took shape. I merged onto the highway with the windows rolled down. The roar outside muffled the chatter in my mind.

Halfway back to the office, a massive church appeared on the right side of the road. I should stop in; they might be expecting me. Would they know my name? Whether or not I stopped to walk through their front doors, each step was predestined at the dawn of time. A reckless car stole my attention as I came to the exit, and I missed the turn.

Instead of trying to ram into my side, a grungy, red, rust bucket of a car flew up ahead and ripped the wheel to the right trying to slam the car in front of me. With a last-second wheel jerk, the car managed to escape by inches. Why would someone provoke an accident in broad daylight, and what did the person in front of me do to warrant the reckless behavior? Again, he shot into our lane, causing the car in front and me to slam on our brakes and cut right. As he sped off, I realized he wasn't after the car in front. He was after me.

I took my spot in the slow lane with shaky hands. Two more times, the same vicious style of attack was attempted right in front of me. By the last time, I could see an invisible force preventing collisions and clearing the way.

Making it back to work unscathed, I wanted a few moments to shake the chaos off. No such luck, though. I was called to the boss's office when I walked through the front door. If they only knew what I had been through this morning. I took my time through the narrow hallway and down the stairs. To my surprise, both bosses were sitting there as I was told to shut the door behind me. This wasn't a good sign. As the conversation ensued, their words didn't quite make it all the way to my ears. They melted and fell short like rolling orbs of color in a lava lamp. My words met theirs in the middle, and I slammed my dead watch on the table for proof as I told them about my lunch journey.

"I'm done here. Fire me if you want, but I'm going back to work now," I said, dismissing myself from the room. The rest of my day was spent trying to make sense of everything in my dusty cubicle and wondering what came next. This was the first outburst I had ever had at work. They were probably in as much shock as I was.

The animosity of the day released its nasty grip as I arrived home and dropped my things at the door. My wife greeted me with random questions. "Honey, what happened to the metal sign in the garage? Did you throw it away? He spent a lot of time making it for you."

She was right. He had made it out of love, and we had been friends forever. There was no way it was carrying anything evil. He made it out of the kindness of his heart, and love is greater than evil.

"Not at all," I said. "I'd never throw it away. One of the screws it was hanging on wasn't right, so I took it down. In fact, I was going to get it from the truck when I got home. I just forgot." I grabbed my keys and headed back out the door. The lowered tailgate revealed both signs and the toy cannon. *Good thing the sign didn't get trashed today; my friend would have never spoken to me again.* I placed the metal sign on the floor below where it once hung. This was a setup the whole time. The enemy was trying to destroy my friendship. Not to mention I was going to trash the one thing my father gave me. To top it all off, I had a stolen sign from work in the back of my truck. Removing the cannon, it went back to its place on the corner shelf. The wood sign would have to wait until tomorrow. I hoped the police wouldn't come for it.

Sleep was a fleeting memory at this point. In the darkness of night, while everyone else's mind drifted away from consciousness, mine desperately tried to unwind the fragile threads between this world and the next. Both worlds seemed to exist hand in hand with nothing but a fragile veil separating us from angels and demons. The silence of my thoughts was interrupted by the backdoor jiggling. *It's not real,* I told myself. With a pop, the door swung open. Maybe I was wrong. The sound of rushing feet flooded the kitchen and reverberated to the bedroom. Why were they here? Who were they here for? Clenching my eyelids shut as the sounds dissipated, I knew they must be heading for the kids' rooms on the other end of the house. This wasn't a robbery. They weren't here for any money. This was a tactical team. My faith was being tested. Even if I had a weapon, going after them would put matters into my own hands and prove my faith was in myself and not God.

The thought that I couldn't run and save my children was clawing at my flesh. If I moved, they would kill us all. Moving back through what sounded to be our living room, the steps of a few men now sounded closer to ten as they overturned furniture and ransacked the house. One broke from the rest of the pack and worked his way to our room. The clicking of his gun against the body armor grew louder as he breached the doorway. He was laden with heavy gear by the sound of it. The grenades on his vest rattled with each strategic step. Cautious and calculating, he moved about the room searching for something. The sound of the others retreating out of the back door drew his attention as he hurried to follow suit. I'm not sure what they came for, but how the air in the room shifted as someone hovered over me in the dark is ingrained in me forever. Staring at the ceiling until daybreak was enough to make a man go mad, but nothing was worth risking the lives of my family. What if they left a lookout to test my faith?

CHAPTER 5

The alarm beeped, and I bolted to the living room to assess the damage. Nothing, not a single thing, was out of place. All those people were running through and tearing up our house. It was like nothing ever happened. Instead of cleaning up and trying to explain last night's intrusion to the wife, I could focus on the day at hand.

The workday was slotted to be full of manager meetings. As a company, we had never done anything like it before. Managers from other locations would descend on our central office, and I was unprepared. There was no itinerary, no bullet points, and nothing to prepare with. I grabbed my brown leather Bible and green highlighter and walked out the door. After all, I couldn't show up empty-handed.

When I backed into the parking lot at work, the wooden sign in my truck bed was screaming to be set free. I had almost forgotten the weathered symbol of fear riding around with me. I grabbed a permanent marker out of the console. I knew what I had to do. It's what Jesus would do. He would hit it head-on with love. The back side of the sign offered a clean slate, a fresh start, and plenty of room for the word *LOVE* to be scribbled in black marker.

The letters filled the space clear to the edges after going around and around, making them as bold as possible. There was, however, enough room to write John 14:6 really small in the top right corner. Someone was sure to see the small verse and be intrigued enough to look it up. The way it had torn from the wall a few days before meant there was no chance of hanging it back up. The base of the stone column marking the entrance was the perfect spot to ensure all who entered would see it. I hoped they would remember to look for love if they lost their way.

My phone smacked the desk as I pulled the Bible and laptop from my bag. One quick run-through on emails, and then the rest of the day could be focused on meetings. Nothing new in the inbox, but the junk mail was exploding. Our website inquiry forms went there, but seeing more than a handful daily was rare. Something told me not to look, but it was part of my job and not a choice. A simple click revealed what my gut already knew. Email after email of nothing but spam, but why so many? Scrolling down further, these were all from the same sender. The writing was a combination of symbols and letters I had never seen before. Each email went on forever. Cyberattack. I wasn't sure who, but someone had tried to breach our security. We were compromised, but I knew who the first meeting needed to be with.

Jumping up, Bible in hand, it was time to prepare. My boots hit the conference room carpet as the lights kicked on. Pausing at the doorway, I stared at the contrast between the nice clean carpet and the filthy boots on my feet. It seemed reasonable at the time to leave my boots outside the door. Cleanliness is next to godliness, and I wasn't letting any filth in. The floor was much softer than I expected for a commercial-grade carpet, but still not the soft fluffy kind from home. I stood in the doorway, my hand on the long credenza. It looked like natural wood, the same as the one on the opposite wall, but both were plastic. What a shame they weren't made from natural wood, the purest material on earth. Tracing my fingers along the fake plastic grooves led halfway down the wall. Everything in the room was deceiving, but I had never noticed. How did I miss something this obvious?

The table centered in the room was stone but looked like wood. The credenzas on both sides were plastic but looked like wood. Even the frames of the mirror behind me and the bluebonnet picture in front of me looked like wood. The lifelike image of bluebonnets was always behind my head because of where I sat. I had never examined it to see if it was a painting or a photograph. With eyes locked in place, my being was pulled toward the picture. From across the room, the tops of the bluebonnets began to sway as if kissed by a gentle breeze. The entire field was slow dancing by the time I was close enough to grasp the entirety of what I was seeing. It was nothing more than a print on canvas, but it was so alive and beautiful.

The plastic frame imprisoned the radiant field, swaying melodically to a light spring breeze. Reaching for the edge, my fingers confirmed the cheap plastic frame and shifted to the canvas. They followed the canvas up the side of the picture as a small green light flashed in the sky. It was calling like a lighthouse in the distance. Reaching for it like a child trying to touch a firefly, I was slow and careful—but too late. The light was gone, swallowed by the sunset.

Turning to the table, I took my seat facing the doorway. Looking down at my Bible, the neon green highlighter clipped to the front reminded me of Mantis, our IT company. Their logo was the same color as the highlighter. I was sure they would be on their way if God wanted their meeting to happen first.

My eyes tracked the direction the highlighter was pointing, and it sent my eyes into the showroom. A large metal rack holding wood fireplace mantles stood against the far wall. A wooden American flag boasting bright red, white, and blue paint spanned the top shelf. Below it lay a dark, rustic beam with baseball-sized holes at each end. It looked like the horizontal piece of a cross, with gaping wounds from spikes. I stared through the door at it each Monday, but I'd never seen it for what it was: the balance between church and state.

It has been about balance since the dawn of time. The

balance between night and day, summer and winter, good and evil. Kings and priests were the original balancers of church and state. Kings are kings because they must get dirty from time to time. Some struggle with this because they desire to be holy, like the priest. However, the best kings in history accepted their roles and went to war. When they kept their priests close and sought God's wisdom and direction, they ruled over illustrious kingdoms and acquired great wealth. Most people nowadays view this relationship as the church and the government or even church and business. I saw the need to balance kings and priests within each company, church, and government. In industry, someone leaning more toward the priest position could never make some of the most challenging decisions. They can't get in the mud like a king can. It's not their fault; they weren't created for it. Kings, on the other hand, run at danger head-on and sleep like babies at night. I could see the roles playing out here in our company. I couldn't believe it had been in front of me this whole time.

Speaking of making decisions, it was time to see who was coming with us if we were about to start building The Way. It was time to begin thinning the herd. Leaving the comfort of the carpet, I marched bootless to the Human Resources desk. Leaning in as Kim typed away, I asked her to write the names of those who weren't at work with an unexcused absence. The list had to be written in pencil, and everyone who made the list was to be let go. Perplexed, she nodded in agreement. I knew we needed people we could rely on when the world collapsed. I was sure it wouldn't be long before all we had was pencil and paper after all the pens ran out of ink and electricity stopped flowing through the powerlines.

With one task down, I returned to the conference room, pants curling under my feet. One of my favorite warehouse guys came down the hall as I hit the doorway, and I motioned for him to come over. "Bring that mantle into the conference room for me, please," I said when he got closer so I could point to it. Before I could sit down, he was already back and wrestled it through the door. We propped the mantle against the plastic credenza. It brought a real piece of God's creation to the room. It was comforting, like having a piece of the cross next to me. Most people viewed the cross as the end, but it was the first step of another miracle. I grabbed the neon highlighter from my Bible and sat down. The IT guys hadn't yet shown up. Maybe they weren't the first meeting after all.

This was the moment my delusions cranked into high gear without letting loose. Until then, they were like safety flares shot from boats in movies, propelled violently skyward in a burst of color, but fading with the same quickness. At this point, I wondered if the president was about to walk in the door or, better yet, *What if I was supposed to be the next president?* Perhaps the powers that be had heard about the giant lifeboat we were about to build.

I had drifted off while planning the future when a coworker popped in, notebook in hand. "You're not in the first meeting," I said as he turned the corner.

"Yes, I am. That's what I was told anyway."

"It changed. You're in the next one. I'm waiting for our store managers, HR, and accounting. The sooner you get them in here, the sooner we'll be done, and we can have the next one," I said with my hands resting on the Bible.

His furrowed brow spoke for itself as he huffed off. I was flipping through the New Testament killing time when everyone started rolling in. Kevin, the manager of our southern location sat at the head of the table to my left.

I motioned to the other manager to sit opposite him. They didn't know it, but I saw the balance. To my left was a king who wasn't scared to come out swinging and get his hands dirty. At the opposite end of the rectangular table sat a priest. He was farther along than he realized. No one in this company was as good at building people up as he was. God, at some point, would reveal it to him. On my right was our young accountant. Much like a king, he worked in the world of numbers, black and white. There was always an answer to be had in his eyes, but not a spiritual one. Across from him, our HR manager, Kim, found her seat last. Much like a priest, her heart was for people, and she searched for the heart of God more than anyone I knew. The table was balanced, except for the empty seat across from me. Someone was missing.

Of course: our dispatcher. "Can someone go grab the dispatcher?" I asked.

I had emailed the group about the Daniel test a week prior so we could review it during the meeting. In Daniel 6, King Darius was tricked into creating a new law to trap Daniel. Daniel's coworkers were jealous of how perfect he was in the king's eyes and wanted him gone. When Daniel refused to follow this new law, they quickly brought it to the king. Distraught, for an entire day the king tried as hard as he could to find a way around the eminent punishment he was supposed to impose on Daniel. With no way out, his favorite appointed official was thrown into the lions' den the following day.

The priests in the room should have known God would protect Daniel from the lions. I wanted the priests to learn from Daniel's perspective. Never back down in their faith, even in the face of danger. I wanted my kings, on the other hand, to see it through King Darius's eyes. With power comes great responsibility. Establishing new rules and regulations in business may harm someone they know and trust if not guided by godly principles. Most importantly, I wanted to know: would they fight for someone they cared about even if the crowd was against them?

The dispatcher came in and sat down across from me. We both walked a fine line, balanced between both king and priest—able to get down in the trenches but also walk close to God. The dispatcher was excellent at fighting in the trenches. Still, he couldn't see God's love yet and how He wanted to use his life for something extraordinary.

I broke the room's silence with a prayer, then jumped right in. "I'm not sure what managers meeting was supposed to happen with who, but you are my managers. A perfectly balanced room. We are the decision-makers, so where do we start?" I asked, looking around the room.

As they spoke about vacation time and hourly pay, the fundamental topics of this type of meeting, all I heard was "not enough." This never-enough mentality had been corroding our culture at an alarming pace, and it was a lie straight from the enemy. Never enough time, never enough money, never enough, never enough. I sliced my way into the conversation to keep from drifting off.

"Hold on, guys," I said. "All I keep hearing is there's not enough. Not enough manpower, not enough resources, not enough time off. So, this is what we're going to do. We'll sell the location out west and bring those employees to our main location. By condensing the two, we should have plenty of what you think we lack. Besides, when we bought the store from its previous owner, their family curse came with it."

They didn't realize this was my first step toward bringing everyone to our corporate office. This was the safest location when the end of the world began. With more people here, we would be able to protect the heart of the company. Besides, I knew for a fact that the new metal roof blocked radar and satellite feeds, so we couldn't be spied on. We would operate undetected.

The stunned look on the managers' faces said it all. What made perfect sense to me confused some and worried others. I chalked it up to their lack of faith and spiritual gifting.

I then dismissed the two youngest in the room so we could talk deeper. They exited the room, and since they were across from each other, the table was still balanced. We went through several more rounds of trying to walk out of this store closure, but they weren't on board yet. We wasted enough time on the topic, so I dismissed the king on my left. Even though this threw the table out of balance on the surface, I was strong enough in spirit to sit across from the remaining two. I motioned to the manager on my right to sit next to the dispatcher across from me. "You two are both ex-military," I said. "This morning, we received a cyberattack on the company. It's bigger and far more advanced than anything I have ever seen. The others won't understand, but I need you both to be alert, watching for threats. This is the first wave of attacks. At some point today, our IT guys should be here to see how bad the situation is. I can't go into more detail, but now I must speak to the dispatcher alone."

The last manager exited the room. This could have been the Daniel test the whole time. He was the last man standing and the one I had to save from the lions' den. I reached across the table and asked if we could pray together. He nodded in agreement, and I launched into a prayer to rip his soul from the grasp of the lion's claws.

We broke from the intense prayer and rolled back in our chairs. My eyes blurred from the pressure squeezing my head like a sponge. The door behind him was a haze, and I followed as he stood and turned for the doorway before his outline faded. Dizziness pushed me against the wall while sliding my boots on. A few feet from the conference room, the office shifted from a looming haze back to the vibrant heart of our company. Whether spiritually attacked or drained from the prayer, I needed some fresh air. Walking by Kim's desk on the way to the back door, she motioned to me.

"Everyone was here today except one person," she said, waving the paper in hand. "He had a family emergency."

I can't fault him; family comes first here. "Great, looks like everyone goes with us," I said in stride toward the back door.

When other companies fell apart as the economy collapsed, we would be a haven for those God sent our way. We would grow in size and prominence as we built The Way and not only have the largest church in the country but the largest business as well. This was how God wanted to bless us, his faithful children. I was certain of it.

These insights warmed my spirit as much as this mid-morning sun on my face. The fresh air had never smelled so wonderful, even sprinkled with diesel fumes from the morning rush of contractors. I walked the loop through the rock yard and back. I smiled at the guy busy loading customers in front of the warehouse. I couldn't help but think of how I made it safe for them as I walked across the only paved section of the loading area. The slight breeze carried the sound of occasional bangs of heavy pallets being loaded on trucks.

Staying to the right took me along the side of the

property neighboring the large tree farm. Rows and rows of trees shot off into the distance. It was almost comical.

I had never seen the balance of the two properties. Walking between two rows of stone led to the edge of the property. All the trees swayed in the soft breeze. They grew from the ground, from good soil. All the while, below the surface, He was forming the stone that rested on the pallets surrounding me. Above and below, the soft swaying leaves and the dense, rigid rock. He, indeed, has provided everything to meet the needs of everyone. I liked how they kept their trees planted in the soil until it was time for a new home. Our stone, in contrast, was bound by wire, rusting over time. It seemed unnatural to bind something made by the hand of God, but it was somewhat symbolic. Long after the wire rusted and fell apart, the stone would still be what God created it to be, much like us. When our bodies fell apart and no longer contained our souls, our spirits would be what God created them to be, free from the limitations of their cages. The low rumble of a passing truck pulled my attention, and my feet, back to the task at hand. I had to finish the loop and get inside for the next meeting.

The first person back to the conference room, I set my boots by the door and was ready to go. The manager of the store I wanted to close stuck his head in the door. Perfect timing. "Come on in, sit down," I said, waving him in. "My phone is on the desk out there. I need you to turn it on and go through all the emails and texts. The ones dealing with the business you handle. Any matters of the heart you bring to me."

With a puzzled look, he said, "Yeah, got it."

I wasn't expecting him to comprehend what was going on. He didn't see the world as I now could. Instead of an explanation confusing him more, I tried to open his eyes to the importance of balance. "The meeting we had earlier was perfectly balanced," I explained. "The next one will look out of sorts, but a balance can be found, even if it's not easily seen. In the next meeting, I want you to look for the angles. We all balance each other out. Look for the angles if you don't see balance across from you. It may be hidden, but it's there."

Looking at me with a blank face, I could tell he didn't get it yet, but he would soon enough. "Now go check my phone, please, and keep me posted," I said, motioning for him to go.

The next meeting was about to start, and the room filled quickly. The table had room for six chairs, and the two extras shoved in the corners were also used. Kim was going to lead this one. She entered last, juggling a handful of papers and a laptop. Projecting her computer to the big screen, she kicked off the meeting. Slide after slide, her nerves calmed as she went along. I watched as my manager's eyes searched for balance in the room. They were both doing an excellent job of stepping out of their comfort zones. This meeting was all about business or the world's view. The one I had held earlier was about the spirit or heavenly view. There was a balance for everything, even the day's meetings.

At the close of the second meeting, it was time for another lap outside. Electricity was pulsing through my veins, and I could barely concentrate long enough to throw my boots on and head for the exit. Launching through the back door, I almost flew by the manager of our southern store as he was lighting his cigarette.

"Let's walk around the loop," I said in stride.

As we walked and talked, the drags on his cigarette

became as deep as the look of concern in his eyes. Pausing the conversation to hug one of the yard workers, I couldn't figure out what he was worried about. Rounding the bend at the back of the stone yard, the office came into view, and out it flew. He let loose with a flick of his cigarette butt and a deep sigh.

"We can't close down a store location. It doesn't make any sense," he belted out.

"I didn't say that at all," I replied, stopping to hug another yard worker. Resuming the walk, his hands pounded the air with the same intensity as his words. "You said we had to close the store multiple times in front of everyone, and it doesn't make any sense."

His words echoed in my ears, piercing through a void where reason and thought once connected words with sentences. "I don't remember. Words are hard for me sometimes," I muttered, straining to piece the conversation together.

I didn't know why I couldn't remember conversations from earlier in the day or why everyone around me seemed confused or concerned. I was the happiest I had ever been and more concerned with making sure everyone felt loved than remembering pointless work meetings.

In silence, we arrived at the back door where our walk had begun, and I fled to the empty conference room. Laying my head down on the Bible, I wondered how many more meetings we would have. I thought if I pretended to sleep for a while, maybe they would cancel the rest. Too wired to sit still, it wasn't long before I was staring at the big wooden flag in the showroom. Shifting my eyes from the flag to the wooden mantle, leaning against the credenza, my head shot up in revelation. Balance was staring me in the face again. The cross-looking chunk of wood and the good old American flag. Balance of church and state. Why didn't I see this earlier? Maybe I wasn't supposed to be a pastor and lead The Way after all. Perhaps I was supposed to be the first prophetic Christian to hold office as the United States president. What better way to change the world? The conference room would make a fine campaign headquarters. We could hang the mantle underneath the television and replace the whiteboard on the opposite wall with the flag. The balance would be restored to the world, and this would be its birthplace.

Later that night, I rolled back through the day's excitement, and it pushed sleep further and further from my grasp yet again. There was too much to plan. Was I supposed to be a pastor or the president? Or was I supposed to be both at the same time? The hours churned away as my thoughts and plans tossed about like tiny leaking boats struggling to stay afloat.

The storm raged on until my eyes found a beacon of hope in a little blinking light on the ceiling. The small, green flash of the smoke detector light in the darkness calmed my brain like a lighthouse beckoning a ship. As my thoughts began to quiet with the blinking rhythm, the pattern was shattered by a piercing red flash. Eyes widened, and now sitting in bed, the light flashed green. Unable to pull my eyes away, I counted seven green flashes. Number eight painted the ceiling with a blood-splatter red.

The tactical team crashed our house last night to bug it. That's why they were here. They planted cameras and wiretapped our home. My flesh wanted to grab a ladder and rip it from the ceiling, but my spirit wouldn't let me. If I did, it would be taking matters into my own hands instead of allowing God to have control. What did they want with my family? What were they after?

CHAPTER 6

I arrived at work, and the overwhelming pressure of seeing through the veil, protecting our house, and working my day job was twisting me like a dry sponge. Unable to turn on the computer, the blank monitor reflected my hollow stare. Coworkers came by to tell me this or ask me that, but my attempts to write down notes ground to a halt. Half sentences faded out, littering the notepad before me. I nodded, deflecting the questions, and forced an, "I'll get back to you," reply. I thought my spirit was taking control of my body, leaving my mind incapable of processing simple worldly tasks. Letters and numbers no longer had meaning. I wondered how I had gotten there. Not only how had I gotten to this point in my life, but also how I had gotten to work.

It was time for a walk and some fresh air. This was too much all at once. I thought I understood what operating in the spirit was supposed to be like, but I had no idea what sacrifices would have to be made. After constant spiritual attacks, now my physical body no longer functioned. I knew if God was in control, it was all supposed to be happening, but what else would this cost me? What did it all mean, and where was this going? Question after question pounded my spirit while I wandered through the stone yard and threw my hands up in frustration at God. My reality was being stolen. An internal war between faith and fear was taking hold where the innocent curiosity of a connection with God once ruled.

Almost back to the office with no more clarity than before the walk started, the internal struggle was thrown aside. Not twenty feet ahead was a group of customers, eight or nine guys deep, circling around a single person. It was hard to count the exact number by how they swayed and jerked like hungry dogs waiting to be fed. Gravitating toward the commotion, they were all gripped by a trance.

Inches behind one of the guys, none acknowledged my presence. I peered between swaying heads and was met with a half-cocked smile and the flash of a snake's tongue from the ringleader. Dead silence hit as his hollow black eyes locked with mine, and all the heads snapped in my direction. Startled and stumbling back a step, I could see all their faces were emotionless and marked with the same cold, hollow stares. The puppet master in the middle had them under control, and the smirk on his clammy face was daring me to make a move.

I lunged forward to smash through the outer circle at him, but he didn't flinch. The stench from his fanged smile set fire to my eyes as his forked tongue flicked about. Reaching for a handshake with my right hand and his shoulder with my left, his face turned from cocky to confused. As I grasped his hand and told him, "Jesus loves you," the color returned to his eyes and cheeks, and the surrounding crowd was released from his clutches.

With the group of customers smiling and free, I could head back inside. No answers fell from the sky, but at least something got done. When I returned to the office, the vice president asked me to join him in the conference room. A manager was already seated and waiting for us. I thought I was in for another day of meetings. I didn't have time or patience, but I obliged and sank into the chair at the end of the table. The VP followed, swinging the door shut, then sat across from me at the head of the table. The weight pressing down on their shoulders conveyed something was wrong. The three of us were close friends, and I had never seen this level of concern on their faces before.

Leaning in, elbows on the table, the VP broke the silence. "I'm not sure what's happening, but we're here to help. Do you know how many loads of material you have coming in next week?"

It was not a question I didn't understand. I was in charge of purchasing and freight for the entire company. But searching for any memory of work duties from the days prior proved to be a task beyond reach. Unable to respond, my chest tightened as the air around me thickened.

"It's okay if you don't remember. We're here for you; don't worry. Did you bring your laptop today?"

I nodded in agreement and barely edged out a, "Yes," between gasps. The manager left the room to retrieve my computer. The deterioration of my mind was now eating away at my emotions. What began as a small nibble here and there was now tearing at the final shreds of normalcy

I had left to lose.

When he returned with the laptop and my notebook, the manager sat next to the VP and slid him my notebook. With scrunched eyebrows, the manager mumbled, "I can't read any of his writing."

"What's your password so we can check purchase orders for this coming week?" the manager asked compassionately.

The question echoed, but my attention was on the bluebonnet picture on the wall. I wished I were there, walking through the field, hand gliding across the tops of the thick, swaying bluebonnets. Nothing between heaven and me except the fiery orange and yellow sky.

"Your password, do you remember it?" ripped me back inside the room. Without words, the air was once again snatched from my lungs with such force my face almost smashed my knees as wailing sobs filled the room. I couldn't respond, because I didn't remember the password or anything else hardly.

"It's okay. We'll figure it out. Everything's going to be all right," one of them said, attempting to console me.

Doubled over with my head buried in my hands and

tears rolling down my face, I couldn't help but wonder, after all I'd been through, was this what would break me? I did not want to look either of them in the eyes, so my hands guided my face to a resting spot on the table. As the last of the emotional rush filtered out, the silence of the room drew my face out of hiding. The chairs were empty, and only my cryptic notepad and locked laptop were left behind. They'd be back soon, but curiosity brought me to my feet. *What's on the notepad?* I didn't remember what I wrote. The words might be written in a code only I could decipher. With spiral notepad in hand, none of it made any sense. Each line started with letters that should make words, but I couldn't make them out. By the end of the line, they faded to squiggly lines like a toddler trying to sign their name.

Like fall leaves in a windstorm, my physical mind was being ripped away in a thousand directions at once. Each gust tore away another thought or memory and crippled my ability to function in this sophisticated environment. Setting the notebook down, I sank into the chair, and the painting called me again. Little yellow flowers sprinkled throughout the bluebonnets were glowing and flashing like lightning bugs on a warm summer night. This was the first time I'd noticed them in the painting. The sky's reflection illuminated the face of the water as it rippled with the breeze. It flickered at first, then sparked into a roaring fire as the sky flashed in a rage. I sat in awe as the sky melted and ran down the picture, spilling over the frame like a candle held to a blowtorch.

The quick snap of the door beside me ripped my attention to the other side of the room. It was one of the company's founders. Could he see the picture melting? His focus was on me, not even a glance toward the wall. He couldn't see it. He sat beside me and looked concerned like the others. "I think we need to get you to a doctor today. Do you have one you go to?" he asked.

It didn't make sense why he wanted to send me to the doctor for no good reason.

"I do, over in Lake Worth," I said, not wanting to give him a name.

"Well, who is it?" he asked. Round and round we went until he dragged it out of me, then left to have someone make the appointment. If everything happened for a reason, maybe I was supposed to go to the doctor.

The manager and vice president made their way back into the room. This time, the newest member of our IT company joined the group. Why did they send the new guy? I wondered. I had only seen him around a few times. Was it possible he had infiltrated their company to get to me? Conspiracy theories swirled in my head. I wondered if he was here to plant fake evidence against me to stop me from running for office or becoming one of the nation's leading pastors. Who was he really working for?

Looking back at the bluebonnets on the wall, they had put themselves back together.

"Good morning," I cheerfully said to the stranger invading my computer.

"Good morning," he repeated, shifting his focus toward me as his fingers stopped piercing the keys. The slow rotation of his head revealed the hollow diamond eyes I had become familiar with. It would have given me chills if I wasn't already shivering because of the cold. A smirk emerged as he finished his response revealing a mouth full of sharp teeth as his forked tongue snapped back in time to not be severed. The glasses on his face acted as magnifying glasses pulling me through his hollow eyes and into the emptiness that used to hold a human soul. My computer meant nothing; I must save the person snatched from this body.

I had to show the evil spirit who was boss and that he couldn't shake me. I had brought my lunch, with fresh-cut fruit in it. If God prepares a table before my enemies, I wanted to see how this one reacted to God's candy being eaten before him. I rushed to grab the fruit from my lunch box and the framed family photo from my desk. I returned and placed the picture between me and the evil spirit controlling the IT guy. His tongue flicked with a hiss as he typed away, taunting me with his slimy grin. The picture between us was the only thing to keep me from taking the spiritual battle to the physical realm.

I peeled the top off the plastic fruit container and ate each bite slowly and methodically, waiting for his response. Nothing, not even a wince from my combatant. "Do you think those bluebonnets are blue? They look violet to me," I said, trying to provoke some interaction.

"I guess they could be either," he hissed back.

"And that beautiful sky. Is that a sunrise or sunset?" I asked, crunching on a grape and pressing him harder.

I knew he wouldn't want to talk about God's creation for long before cracking.

"Could be either, I suppose," he growled.

"You know," I fired back, "my daughter loves sunsets, but I love sunrises. Both are beautiful works of art. Wouldn't you agree?"

He cut his eyes at me and, with a finger, pushed his glasses back up the bridge of his nose. "I suppose," seeped through his jagged teeth and slithered through my ears, piercing the depths of my spirit.

I needed some air, and the room was too cold to take anymore.

"I'll be back," I said, jumping to my feet and already halfway through the doorway.

Outside, I hoped the sun would pull the chill from my bones as I walked to the side of the property bordering the tree farm. Row after row of beautiful trees with blazing green leaves pulled me in. Birds hopscotched from one limb to another. The joy restored warmth to my soul as I strolled up and down perfect rows of adolescent trees. A cool breeze floating through the leaves provided a hypnotizing backdrop and drowned out the noise of the morning. I wanted to walk among the trees forever in God's masterpiece, but it was time for me to go home.

Back inside, I peeked into the conference room, and it looked like they didn't need me here, getting in the way, anymore.

"You have a doctor's appointment later today, and one of us will take you." said the vice president. "Are you hungry yet? I'm going to grab us some lunch in a minute."

"Sounds good," I replied, pulling my head out of the doorway. It was time for me to sneak out; the quicker, the better. Snatching the keys from my desk, I bolted. Turning the corner to the showroom that led to the front door, I stopped in my tracks. The founder was standing on the other side of the glass doors, arms crossed, talking to someone. I had to escape out of the back door, or he would stop me. I'd have to go by him to get to my truck, but there would be enough distance so he couldn't get to me.

Walking with intensity, one notch from a sprint, I breached the corner at the front of the building. It was now or never, and I wasn't looking back for anything.

"James! Hey, James!" screamed the founder as I flew by. Dust was kicking up from the gravel and lingering like smoke trails from my shoes. They had caught me. The founder and the manager were not more than ten feet behind me.

I jumped into the driver's seat and kept my hand on the door so I could slam it shut if they tried to grab me and asked, "What do you guys want?"

The founder shouted, "I want you to stay."

I wasn't sure if his tone was nervous or angry, but I didn't want to stick around for small talk.

"Well, I want to go," I shouted back.

"We have to take you to your doctor's appointment here in a little bit," chimed in the manager.

"I didn't make a doctor's appointment. He did," I said, pointing toward the founder.

With an emotional breakdown coming on strong, I looked at the manager and, as calmly as possible, said, "I want to leave now."

I knew they cared about me like we were family, but I didn't understand why they were trying to keep me there.

"We'll let you leave if you go straight to your doctor. You'll be early, but at least you can take your time and be careful," pled the manager.

Bingo: there was my way out. "Yeah, I remember where it is. I'll head there now."

I didn't intend to go and slammed the door to my freedom.

I left the parking lot, but the first red light stalled my getaway. I wasn't mad about it, though. I had never seen a red light with such depth of color. It was a radiant beacon glowing like the hot coals of a roaring fire. A brilliant emerald-green burst forth in a flash as a car pulled up on the right. Inching my wheels forward, the tinted driver's window slid down. When it reached its resting point, the head of the driver rotated my direction. It was a coworker with jet-black hair and eyes to match. His hand pegged the bottom of his chin, and with the vigor of a possessed man, he displayed the sign of the devil while violently lashing his tongue out. The honk from the car behind brought me back to the task at hand, driving. It wasn't real. It couldn't have been him; the car was gone.

Cutting through the side streets to the highway was always my route. I had never noticed how brilliant the colors were lining the concrete forest. From the signs on the businesses to the billboards, even down to the cars on the road, the world was alive with vibrant, dancing colors. The scales had been removed from my eyes, and I could now see the world in its full glory.

I made my way to the highway, and a small black dot in the rearview mirror grew to the point I could make out a tail. Someone was following me. It wasn't a chase. They would have had me by now. This is what they were trying to protect me from. They knew someone was after me. I wondered if someone was supposed to meet me at the doctor's to inform me what was happening. I was heading in the opposite direction, though. I had to make it home. The heat was on, and I knew I had to baptize myself again for protection. The black dot, now bigger in the mirror, had turned into an SUV. My sweaty hands gripped the wheel. I could gas it and run, or act like I wasn't scared. Running wasn't an option, not for me. If God was in control, even if this car ran me off the road, it's what God intended to happen. I was sure of it. As my heartbeat slowed, the blacked-out SUV sped by on the left. I knew then I had to have more faith and less dependence on my reasoning.

I had changed into swim trunks and made it a few

feet from the back door when my wife's voice rang out behind me.

"What are you doing home?" she shouted as I opened the door.

"Because I came home," I barked back, leaving the door wide open behind me. I was down the stairs and throwing my towel on a lawn chair before she made it outside. Nothing was going to stop me from baptizing myself, not even her. I plunged into the icy swimming pool and began praying while dunking myself under the water in every direction possible. I had never done this before; it had to be done right. My wife was waiting when I emerged from the icy water.

"What are you doing at home? You never leave work early," she asked in a panic.

"Too many meetings," I said. "I'm tired of them."

Trying to get past her and back inside, she stepped between me and the door, cranking up the intensity.

"Call Kevin. He'll tell you all about it," I said.

"How am I supposed to call him?" she asked. "You left your phone at work." She was right. I had forgotten all about my cell phone and computer. How did she know?

"I spoke with your work earlier, and they said they scheduled a doctor's appointment for you. Why didn't you go?" she asked, hands on her hips.

"Because they made it for me, and I don't know why they did," I said, trying to find a way around her.

With her close on my heels, I finally made it back inside. She pleaded with me to go to the hospital for blood work. I had no idea why a doctor or hospital was needed and refused repeatedly. After a hot shower and a few hours of begging, I agreed to go. It seemed important to her at the time, but I'd never been a fan of hospitals. They reek of sorrow and sickness.

CHAPTER 7

The glowing cars and fluorescent scenery whipped by the car windows like a psychedelic movie. The raging sea of colors was calmed by the towering hospital's shaded parking lot. The massive stone walls protruding from the flat, cold face of the building hid the setting sun and choked out the last rays of sunshine and color. The hospital's logo—a green glowing medal of victory—caught my eye like a giant beacon of hope. Not just any shade of green, but Mantis green, our IT company. I had no idea they owned an entire hospital, but it made perfect sense. This place must be their playground with all the electronics and gadgets. I knew they were already watching us like guardian angels on the cameras.

Scanning the walls for hidden cameras on our way to

the door, I debated how many bodies hospitals hid versus how many they healed. Almost to the door, I changed directions and bolted for a bright orange port-a-john sitting on the edge of a construction zone across the parking lot.

"Where are you going?" my wife shouted, throwing her hands up.

"I have to pee," I said over my shoulder in stride.

"But there are bathrooms inside."

She was too late. The door latched behind me. They weren't going to make me pee in a cup so they could alter it. I agreed to go, but I never agreed to cooperate. At this point, I was sure they were setting me up so I couldn't become president, but I was ready for a fight.

When I emerged, her tilted head and squinting eyes told me she wasn't in the mood for an explanation. Falling in line behind her, I pulled the bill of my hat down without exchanging words. The heavy sliding glass doors swallowed us whole, cutting off the outside world. We each grabbed a disposable mask as we passed through the second set of sliders into the threshing floor that separated the living from the dead. Packed from wall to wall with sickness, pain, and agony, I bet Death himself cackled at their moans. My wife found a couple open seats against the floor-to-ceiling windows that separated us from the real world. We were stuck, like harmless little fish in a decaying aquarium rotting from the inside out.

The mask over my face did nothing to hold back the stench of the rotting lives surrounding us. Hunched over and gasping for air, I tore it off, hoping to regain my breath while heaving in distress. The air was so thick with pain and suffering that it choked the hope from the room. My distress subsided enough to sit up, and I was met with cries of agony from all directions. Moaning and violent sobs crashed against each other like a raging sea churning against weathered rocks. Echoing off the walls of the sprawling room, the gnawing and gnashing of pain and fear lunged for our spirits.

I scoured the room for a way out, not knowing if the goosebumps on my wife's arms were from lack of heat or Fear sinking its teeth in. A uniformed officer walked by and paused long enough to bark at me to put my mask on before stomping off. A bolt of electricity shot down my spine at his ferocious command.

"I'm out of here. I got to get out. I'll be outside," I said, raising the mask and jumping to my feet.

"Stay right in front of this window so I can see you," my wife said, unable to stop me.

To the right of the doors was a grassy area framed by cold concrete sidewalks. Lined with small bushes and sprays of monkey grass, the site hosted a large, solid block of stone for a bench in the center. It was much warmer out here, and alive, for that matter. I pulled the mask from my face and stuffed it in my pocket. Fresh, crisp air filled my lungs once more as I sat on the bench and looked out over the sea of cars.

The whoosh of the sliding glass doors drew my attention as an officer rushed toward his squad car in the middle of the lot. Our eyes met, his brow wrinkled, his nose scrunched, and I scrambled for my mask as the world slowed to a crawl. Struggling to fish it from my pocket in slow motion, the world broke free, and I could pull it to my face. The officer was almost in his car but still looking toward me with fire in his eyes. I buried my face in my knees and covered my head, fearing he was coming for me. The squad car door slammed shut fifty yards away but cracked like it was next to me. Clutching the back of my head, the siren screeched like a banshee, then silence. I was sure he wanted me to look up so he could shoot me. Not today. I wasn't going to die, not like that. A blast of his horn followed the clap of a handgun. I was trembling, even though I didn't hear a bullet whiz by. Resisting the reaction to jump and run, my head stayed buried. I was frozen.

After enough silence, I heard a conversation in the distance. As I raised my head, I saw the squad car was in the same place, but no cop. Maybe my IT friends were more than business owners. They must be CIA or Secret Service. The gunshot I had heard had to be them getting to the officer before he could strike. They must have had a sniper on the roof, perched and ready. I couldn't be out in the open like this. They saved me once but had too much ground to cover outside. I fished the mask from my pocket, took one final breath, and crossed into the cold pit of despair.

Finding my wife in the same spot, I put my head down and leaned into her side for warmth. With my eyes sealed shut, I began praying in my spirit for the injured souls around us. The words flowing through my mind became a lighthouse in the raging storm. As with any light in the midst of darkness, it beckoned the shadow-lurking creatures. The harder I prayed, the more pain and suffering swirled around us. Fear commanded the room like an orchestra conductor. Wave after wave of his hand stirred the groaning and weeping while he laughed. The weight was too heavy for me to hold. Fear clawed at my skin, searching for a way to attack my soul. I stood, looking for a place to hide, anywhere.

The single-person bathroom was the best place to hide in a panic. The door lock twisted and slid into place with a thud. The room was silent. The torment subsided. I turned to the pedestal sink mounted inches from the door and turned the water on. Both hands clutched the cold porcelain. Slumped over, it supported my weight, and a tear rolled from the tip of my nose. Why me? Why was I the one called to absorb this immense pain and sorrow? I wasn't strong enough on my own. Working up the courage to face myself in the mirror, I raised my quivering chin until the bill of my hat gave way to my bloodshot eyes. I couldn't remember the last time I had looked in the mirror, but the eyes staring back belonged to a worn-out, empty shell of a man. Splashing water on my face to hide the tears, I had to get back to my wife. She wasn't safe by herself.

Before I could sit, she met me halfway. "What took you so long?" she asked, throwing her hands up.

I shrugged my shoulders and followed her to the counter. She pleaded with the nurse at the counter that we'd been waiting too long and needed a room. I was busy surveilling the waiting area. A few cameras housed in little black globes were mounted on the ceiling behind the counter. I was okay waiting for a room, because my buddies were watching. They cleared a path for us to move on to the next challenge. I was sure of it. We were being tested and wouldn't get to the next level until I figured out how to pass each test. A woman opened the wooden door to our left and called my name. We had made it through level one.

We were ushered to the next room, each taking a seat crammed against one another. It wouldn't be long before I got us out of there now that I knew I had to crack the code. A man in scrubs with thick, black-rimmed glasses entered the opposite door and sat at the computer. As he asked questions through his mask, I remained silent, trying to determine if he was a friend or foe. There were no cameras in the room. We were on our own, and my back was against the wall. The only way out was the open door across the room. My wife jumped in and fielded the questions as I inspected the room. Beyond her was a dry-erase board taking up most of the wall. Drawn left to right were vertical columns across the length of the board. Tally marks, letters, and numbers filled the board. It was the code I had to crack to move on.

A nurse walked in and grabbed a marker from the tray. Removing the cap and writing at the top, she blocked my view.

"Is your shift just now starting, or do you get to go home soon?" I asked, excited to take a crack at this new game.

"Just getting started," she said.

I knew she had smiled through her mask because her cheeks tightened, and her eyes lit up. She was on our side. Before I could ask the next question, another nurse appeared beside her.

"Sir, sir," the doctor tried to gain my attention for questioning, but my wife jumped in again. She had my back.

"Is your shift just starting?" I asked the second nurse. The two nurses were now four at the board, each with an eraser in one hand and a marker in the other. They turned in unison, "Just getting started."

Writing and erasing at the speed of hummingbird wings, I couldn't decipher anything while they fought for space. Three nurses were for us, but the fourth was a plant. That's why they were scrambling to jumble and erase the coded messages. They hoped I'd catch the key to escape, but I couldn't.

Feeling defeated, my focus shifted to the doctor in time to hear him say, "We'll get you back out to the waiting room and call you when we get a room freed up."

Tears built in my wife's eyes as she begged for a room. "We can't go back out there," she said. "He can't handle it."

With the last nurse squeezing out of the door, the male intake nurse agreed to find us a room. She got us through to the next level. I wasn't sure how many floors the hospital had, but I knew we had to reach the roof for the Secret Service to pick us up in a helicopter. Shown into another room, we didn't even see the elevator. It wasn't a good sign; we should have been going up.

My wife sat against the wall, rubbing her arms for warmth as I slid onto the frozen sheets of the hospital bed. A small window in the pale steel door allowed prying eyes to glance like we were animals on display. This level appeared more complex to maneuver, more like a jail cell. I hoped my wife could keep her composure so we could keep progressing. With a soft knock and a swift door swing, the doctor's presence filled the room. Friend or foe, I wasn't sure yet. The room was much too dim for reading the intentions in his eyes. He began to ask questions, and I searched the room for clues. I waited for something, anything, to jump out and grab me. At first glance, it looked identical to all the hospital rooms I'd ever been in.

I racked my brain, looking for a way out, and my wife took the lead again. She inundated the doctor with stories of how weird I'd been acting and that I had walked out of work in the middle of the day. People leave work early all the time and don't get escorted to the hospital. I still wasn't sure what all the fuss was for. Demanding a CT scan, she fought against the doctor's initial instinct that I was on drugs. Alarms sounded; she was onto something. He skipped straight to drugs. We couldn't trust him. He wanted to throw us on the street after charting I was on drugs in my permanent file. The media would have a field day. He was setting me up. I needed the blood work done so it was on record I was clean before running my big campaign.

The CT scan would prove my brain was in perfect shape. This was going to turn out in my favor after all. People would have to believe I operated in the spirit and saw behind the veil with a clean bill of health. There wouldn't be any other explanation. It was the perfect way to defend against political attacks. To my wife's relief, he agreed to run the tests and left to submit the orders.

After an eternity of freezing in the colorless icebox, a nurse appeared to draw blood. Not long after, my escort for the CT scan arrived to guide me through the maze of empty hallways. Searching for a way out, the exit signs and elevators had gone into hiding. The tech led us through a door, much like the others, and ushered me in. Politely, he instructed me to lie on the table protruding from the massive machine in the center of the room. I didn't see a reason not to. I'd made it this far. Maybe it would unlock the next level.

With a soft hum, the table slid into the mouth of the slumbering giant. The growl intensified to the roar of a jet engine as the walls whipped around my head like a tilt-a-whirl. Sensations rushed faster than the lights whizzing past my face. My heart pounded, my stomach churned, and my cold, clammy hands clenched the table. What if they were wiping my memories, or worse, implanting new ones? I had to get out before I ended up drooling and staring out of a window for the rest of my life. There was nowhere to run in this endless maze of hallways, and I couldn't leave without my wife. I was seconds away from launching myself out of the mind-melting coffin when the sounds faded. It was slowing to a stop. As we walked back to the room, I searched the far corners of my mind for any gaping holes where memories once lived.

Back with my wife, who was still trembling in the subzero temperatures, I said, "Here, honey, take this blanket." I hoisted the paper-thin cover from the bed before sitting down.

Looking up from her phone with sorrowful compassion, she said, "I'm not shaking because I'm cold. I'm shaking because my nerves are fried."

She went back to typing on her phone, and I lay down, pulling the cover over myself. I knew at any minute we would be escorted to the roof and flown off for the next phase of this cryptic plan God had for us.

Passing the time, I tossed and turned, sat and stood. The suspense was killing me. It should be time to go any minute. By now, it was the middle of the night, and we had the perfect cover of darkness to make our getaway. Another soft knock, followed by the paperwork-wielding doctor. My wife dropped her phone on her lap, and I sat attentively on the bed, both of us excited to get the results.

"His blood work and the CT scan both came back normal. No abnormalities in either," he said with a heavy tone and despairing eyes in my wife's direction.

"That's great news," I said, popping out of bed. "That means I'm good to go."

With a sigh, the doctor turned his sight to me. "What it means is this is more of a mental thing. Physically you are fine, but chemically or neurologically, something isn't functioning as it should. We need to find you some help."

My wife was now on her feet and clung to each word.

Something wasn't right. I knew he was against us. My tests were perfect. This was a setup from the word go.

"How do perfect results equal something is wrong? I've never heard of such a thing. It's time for us to leave," I shouted at the doctor.

"Sir, you're going to have to calm down," he said, raising a shaky hand in defense. "I think we need to do a mental intake on your husband." He looked at my wife.

"I'm sorry," she responded in my defense. "We came straight here, and he hasn't eaten all day. What are the steps for the mental assessment?"

This was ridiculous, but I couldn't leave here without her. The doctor exited, and no begging or pleading would get my wife to go. Not until we did the mental assessment, anyway. Within minutes the doctor returned with two sandwiches in plastic triangle containers and two cans of soda. Setting them down on the table, he informed us the technician would be with us in a few minutes. Inspecting the container, it didn't appear to be tampered with, but I wouldn't put anything past him.

Before finishing the sandwich, a nurse walked in, pushing an iPad mounted on a three-foot pole. "The technician will be with you shortly," she said, rolling it next to the bed and leaving.

Swallowing the last bite of the stale sandwich, I turned to my wife and asked, "What's the iPad for?"

Looking up from her phone with tired eyes, she explained, "It's for the virtual meeting. He's on call, but we're almost done, and then we can go."

More tests and questions to pass for the sole purpose of being told passing meant something must be wrong. I could do this all night if necessary; bring it on.

Out of the darkness, a man appeared on the small screen. What kind of doctor was this? He was sitting at a kitchen table in an apartment. After spouting his credentials, the questions began. Not more than a few questions in, my wife took the lead from me. I was impressed. She was better at this than me. They were trying to entrap me with questions to use all the answers against me later. If she answered them, nothing would hold up, because the answers didn't come from my mouth. We must be in the final round. I bet the Secret Service was as tired of waiting as I was. As quickly as he appeared, the questioning ended, and nothing was left but an empty screen on a stick.

We were going to the next level any minute. We had to have passed. The original doctor returned with papers in hand. I couldn't risk talking to him at this stage. We were too close to the end of this for me to lose my cool and punch him in the face. He handed the paperwork to my wife, and he exited the room as she threw her purse over her shoulder. It was time to go. I wanted to be surprised, so I followed her. After the first hallway, no escort yet. We reappeared in the waiting room, where we had begun, and exited through the front doors. We should have gone to the roof. I wasn't sure what was going on. In disbelief, I tried to understand what had gone wrong as we walked through the parking lot and climbed into the car.

Replaying the events over and over was halted once we reached the road, by the flaming red taillights of the cars in front of us. The lights were much more intense in the dark, and oncoming headlights flew toward us in a blaze of white fire so fierce I needed to shield my eyes as they passed. It wasn't until we reached the country roads closer to home that the light show subsided. Staring into the darkness, the realization that my life was crumbling around me rose up and stole the last thread of courage in my body. Ripping the air from my lungs in giant heaves as tears flowed down my face, Fear had wrapped its gnarled fingers around my stifled being. "It's going to be okay, honey," my wife said, rubbing her hand along my slumped back. "Are you scared?"

"No," I groaned between tears and sobs. "As long as you're with me, there's nothing I'm afraid of." Swimming in tears and confusion, the last tethered shred of hope I had left was not admitting Fear had fractured my spirit.

CHAPTER 8

The rising sun peered through our sheer curtains before I deciphered what the night before had meant. No sleep again, but there was no sense staying in bed any longer. The view would be better from the patio. Still wearing the same clothes from the day before, I pounced out of bed with renewed hope and energy. Every sunrise is a new day and another chance. The concrete deck pierced my feet with a frigid bite, hurling me toward the nearest lounge chair.

I watched the night lose its grip as the sun set fire to the morning sky. It climbed on the backs of the towering trees, revealing the prancing silhouettes of a couple playful squirrels. Tracking them between the puffs of steam rising from my breath, they ran across several skinny trees and down the ancient oak at the fence. Statelier than the other trees, he neither groaned nor creaked when the wind ripped through his branches. I prayed my faith would hold as firm and steadfast to withstand the storms coming my way.

The squirrels fought over fallen acorns as God's still, small voice descended around me. *Do you see those squirrels, my son? They want for nothing. I have provided everything. Do you see that tree, my son? I grew it from a seed, it is mine. Had I told you what it would grow into when I planted it long ago, you would have known before it sprouted. Knowing what it will grow into does not mean it will happen on your time or how you thought it would look.*

Of course, how could I have been so naïve? I was along for the ride and in control of nothing. I knew then it wasn't up to me to figure things out. The sun was now well above the trees, the air had lost its bite, and more tiny creatures had come out to play. Two squirrels had turned into a block party. Barn swallows with bright blue crowns and cinnamon bellies darted through the sky, leaving fluorescent trails like screeching fireworks. The depth of colors swirling about was beyond the reach of description. My extreme joy from such beauty was equally matched by the sorrow that no one could share the experience with me. Even the pink potted flowers around the deck glowed like little neon lights. In awe of their magnificence, my bare feet braved the concrete to venture closer to one of the pots.

With a soft pop, I caressed the petals from underneath and separated flower from stem. I could smell the sweet aroma radiating from this jewel long before it reached my nose. It felt like the first time I'd ever smelled a flower. Feet from my head, an ear-piercing cackle rang out. I shielded my head from an attack, but nothing was in the sky above me. It rang out again from the tree line, straight ahead. From the shadows of a tree hopped a crow as black as night, cackling as if he was laughing at a devilish joke. Like a marching band led by a conductor, another crow joined the mocking, followed by another, then another. From the tops of the trees emerged an army of cackling crows. Their sinister laughing dug into my skull like wolves tearing at a fresh kill.

I held my ground against the pint-sized mockers, attempting to stay calm. They had to have been some sort of messengers or watchmen. The limbs were alive as the crows hopped and clawed to gain a closer position, like the bloodthirsty crowd at an ancient colosseum. Though one perched farther back among the trees and much higher than the rest. He was more significant than the brood below. The ominous silhouette belonged to a wretched old buzzard. He twisted from side to side, offering glimpses of the shriveled crimson head protruding from his skinny little neck. With each low, guttural hiss, the crows hopped and howled with anticipation. The crows were mindless spectators, but the buzzard was the general.

Feeding on carcasses and mayhem, he made a perfect puppet for the enemy. None of the buzzard's henchmen could pass the fence line below the trees. I smirked to myself. It appeared prayers did work, and our property was protected. No sense in taking any chances, though, so I made a few loops around the yard in prayer. The world drew closer with each brittle leaf crackling beneath my bare feet. My spirit was grounded by the soft black soil and tiny wisps of tender grass. Stepping with great care and precision, the ground became a dance floor and my prayers a booming melody. After a few graceful passes of fortifying prayer, the path led back inside without a second thought of cackling crows.

A few hours later, the house was brought to life by the chiming doorbell. What our tiny dog, Cooper, lacked in stature, he made up for with ear-shattering precision when company came calling. Snatching him up as he broke toward the door, I took him to the study as my wife answered. A young man with dark hair, glasses, and broad shoulders stood outside. He was ten feet from the door, hanging back while whomever he was with spoke to my wife. The recessed entry in the porch provided a blind spot where the other man had disappeared. *Must be salespeople. We get them from time to time out here. The bugs, the yard, the solar panels, blah, blah, blah.* With French doors between us, the foyer muffled the conversation.

Our yapping heathen escaped when the front door shut, and he snarled at the older man leaving the entry. With a flat-brimmed boater's hat atop his gray hair and a slight wobble, his short, stocky frame meandered around the corner.

"What did they want?" I asked, flinging the French doors open.

"They're here to clean the concrete haze off the windows. Don't you remember? They called last weekend to set up the appointment," she said with concern.

I knew they had to be here, at this time, for a reason and that I should introduce myself.

Raising the garage door revealed a small, silver, single-cab work truck parked in the driveway with ladder racks. The men met me a few feet past the shadow of the house.

"Hello, sir," said the older gentleman, reaching for a shake. "This is my apprentice, who also happens to be my grandson."

A full head taller than him, his grandson stepped out from behind the plump old man with his hand out. When I reached for his hand, the bright white state of Texas leapt from his shirt. Hundreds of guns, all makes and models, combined to form the Lone Star state. I released his hand and smacked him on the chest several times with a burst of nervous laughter. He flinched and stepped back.

"Nice shirt. I love guns too," I said, realizing they must be here for some sort of protection.

"He's shipping off next week to Hawaii for training," bragged his white-bearded grandfather.

"Training for what?" I asked, turning my attention to grandpa, now making his way to their truck.

Leaving my side, his grandson shrugged and said, "The old man is deaf in one ear. He didn't hear you."

Both men unpacked their equipment, and I returned to the house to unpack my thoughts. The training must be military, but why would he be learning how to wash windows? Something didn't make sense, and they didn't look alike either.

Grandpa made his way around back, and, from the living room couch, I saw him adding water to his bucket through our picture windows. He was alone, and it was the perfect chance to ask questions. I snuck out of the back door while holding Cooper back from attacking.

"How do you get the concrete off the windows?" I asked, coming up on his left side.

He rang out the scrubbing pad, looking up from the bucket of suds. "Elbow grease and my secret solution here. Simple as that," he said with a beaming smile. Working on a small area on the window in front of me, it melted right off.

He checked out, but where was his so-called grandson

lurking around? I set off shoeless around the house, leaving the old man to work. I found the grandson far from where he should have been, cleaning the window to my daughter's room.

"Hey!" I shouted in stride, waving. "What are you doing there?"

Turning toward me, he dropped his squeegee in the bucket. "Cleaning your windows. What are you doing?" he fired back.

"I thought you were only doing the windows around back. What are you doing up here?"

"My grandpa told me to start here, so that's what I'm doing," he said, turning his back to me.

At that point, I put some space between us. From the clumsy way he worked to clean the window, there was no way he was a window washer, not even a beginner. I knew he couldn't be evil either, though. I had walked the yard praying before they showed up. My face felt flush. I had forgotten to go around to the front in prayer. That's why he was in the front, and the old man was around the back. Grandpa was able to walk around back because he was righteous. I put more distance between us, using a slow sidestep so my eyes could keep watch. A brown leather holster hung from his hip. It swung low and appeared too large for a gun. As he walked toward the next window, I saw something heavy rested inside by how it swayed.

Around back, sweet, old grandpa was finishing his first window. It had been months since we could see through the haze, and now it was spotless. He knew what he was doing.

"Looks great. How much for washing all the windows, since your grandson is up front?" I asked.

No response. After repeating myself, I remembered he was deaf in one ear and moved to his good side, causing him to catch my reflection in the window.

"We had a price for the back of the house, not the rest. How much for all the windows?"

Wiping the last little bit with a rag, he smiled. "Same price. All the windows on your house need to be done with this solution," he said with a wink.

The solution was the key. I was convinced it was a shield so evil spirits couldn't enter our home. That's what took him so long to get to us; he had waited until we needed his help. I gave him a respectful nod of thanks and left him to his work.

My wife met me in the kitchen. "Honey, leave them alone while they work," she said.

I was glad she didn't know the truth and passed her with a smile on my way to the bedroom. The curtain didn't keep the light out but would provide a slight level of privacy. Not ten minutes after laying down to wrap my brain around the previous night's adventure and our unexpected guests, a soft scratching noise crawled into bed with me. Thinking the old man was on this window now, I figured they should be done soon at this rate.

The soft sound of a scouring pad on a metal pan gave way to a forceful, quicker grinding. Each pass across the window overtook the previous. I buried my head in the covers, but it did nothing to block out the intensifying echoes pounding against the walls. The volume continued to crank as if rabid cats were scratching and ripping my brain apart from the inside out. Writhing in agony, the shadow in the window caused me to jump out of bed in terror, my hands pinned against my ears. It wasn't the old man, but how did the grandson get past the fence?

Heading toward the living room, my flight mode faded as fight mode kicked in. I shot out of the back door. Landing on the back patio, I hooked a left toward the grandson.

"What are you doing back here?" I fired off, rounding the corner to where he was cleaning.

"Still working," he said, nostrils flaring as he clenched the squeegee.

Our eyes were locked, neither budging.

"Okay then, carry on," I said, backing out of the situation.

I was convinced at that moment that he wasn't at our house to clean the windows. From the look on his face to the shirt covered in guns, I knew he was a killer, not a cleaner.

I backpedaled until I had a far enough head start to get away. The old man caught my eye on the other side of the porch. Seeing my reflection in the window, he turned to greet me.

"I have something for you," he said with a smile. "I think you could use these." Digging into his pocket, he pulled out a closed fist and twisted his palm upward. His weathered fingers unfolded, revealing two copper pennies.

They each had a hole punched in them shaped like a cross. Pushing them around with his thumb revealed the crosses themselves. "These are for protection. Keep them with you," he said, motioning for my hand to dump them in.

Rolling them in my hand while smiling back, I knew what to do. These would add another layer of protection around the house. My prayers for protection hadn't worked so well. I started on the south side of the house and threw a cross at the fence line. Next, I walked to the east side and tossed one of the pennies. The second cross was thrown on the north side for balance and the last penny for the front yard at the street. I had to get back inside. I was too exposed in the front yard, but hopefully the pennies would help.

I sat on the couch and watched through the windows as the young window-washing imposter lugged his bucket and ladder around to the patio. When he began cleaning the first one, he turned at an angle, and his brown leather holster swung between him and the window. Something black and rectangular was lodged in it, with the end hanging out. It wasn't even close to the shape of a gun. Before I could investigate, my skull was racked by an earsplitting shrill, sending me reeling on the couch. After an eternity, the noise released its grip for a few seconds, only to come raging in like a screaming banshee again. My convulsing body was defenseless as I clutched my ears and watched his holster swaying back and forth, taunting me.

Twice as long as the first round, the second wave almost split my head in two before coming to an abrupt halt, so I fled to the bathroom for refuge. Through squinting eyes and a throbbing headache, I checked the mirror for signs of blood seeping from my ears. The dull tapping of my wedding ring on the counter was a pleasant sign that there was no permanent damage. He didn't have a gun in his holster. He was trying to erase my mind with high-frequency sound waves. I'd heard about those experimental government weapons but didn't think they were real. Someone wanted me out of the picture, and his poor grandpa didn't even know the truth. I was no longer safe anywhere. They knew where I lived.

The shower looked like an excellent place to lay low at the time. I figured the running water should muffle any more brainwashing attempts. With the dial cranked too hot, steam filled the large walk-in shower as I returned to the mirror. I stood eye to eye, gazing into the depths of a man I knew pretty well. No secrets between us and nothing to fear. Now a perfect stranger wrought with fear and uncertainty was crumbling before me. Breaking down, piece by piece. The steam billowed out of the shower and crawled up the mirror as my reflection faded to nothingness. Stepping into the shower, my battle-worn body dropped to the floor, weak and trembling, finding rest beside the cascading river of tears.

Every ounce of sorrow drained from my spirit while lying on the tile floor, until I found the strength to sit up. Leaning against the wall, hot water rained on my face like a thousand drums pounding a war cry. *Get it together,* I told myself. I was hiding on the floor while my family was fending for themselves. What if sweet old grandpa was an act, and they stormed the house when they couldn't get me? Drying off in a panic, I bolted to the closet for something to throw on.

Swiping a shirt from a hanger on the rack, the world slammed to a crawl. The shirt crept toward me, and the hanger ticked upward like a watch's second hand reaching its peak before shifting back in the other direction. With a puff, a black haze emanated from a leather book on the shelf like a kindling fire. It drifted around the other books and spilled off the shelf toward the floor. With a crack, the empty hanger smacked the wall, and the haze vanished. I dropped my shirt and grabbed the book.

It was a brown leather-bound journal with a Celtic cross etched on the cover. Opening the first couple of pages, I remembered buying it when I was away at college decades ago. Flipping through the pages, some had words, and others were erratic scribblings and chaotic drawings. I had found the sleeping giant. This was the source of evil spirits terrorizing our home. Slamming it shut, I finished getting dressed and slid the journal into the waistband of my loose shorts. I tied the drawstring to keep it in place.

Taking note while emerging from the bedroom with careful steps toward the back door, nothing looked out of place, and no one spotted me. Outside, the cleaners tossed soaked rags into an empty bucket to the right, so I broke left, pretending to inspect their work. Rounding the corner of the house in stride, I spotted the perfect hiding place until I could burn it later. Sliding the book from my waistband in stride, I tossed it between the hippo-sized propane tank and the four-foot cedar fence it lived behind. My momentum carried me through the gate, over the driveway, and back inside through the garage door without looking back.

A few minutes later, the doorbell rang, setting the dog off. This time, my wife rushed out the door with a checkbook. Bouncing between the wall and the couch like a pinball, I was torn between chasing her or waiting to see if she returned. Fear won. I couldn't stop the pacing. Back and forth, back and forth. My fingers were tugging at my hair, trying to rip the dread from my body. The door swung open, and she emerged with the light at her back. A sense of relief flooded over me as the lock latched into place.

Evening set in. The world came to a crawl, but my mind was still a blazing fire. The pieces to the puzzle were being doused with gasoline and turned to ash before any two could fit together, forming a single thought. My wife lying beside me in the darkness, her hand in mine, was the last anchor point tethering me to this world. Drifting deeper into the hollowness of the night, a distant dragging noise snapped me back to the bedroom. The sound was joined by another as the volume grew. Working closer to the bedroom door, the dragging became a distinct sound of sharp claws dragging across the walls. Cutting into the layers of paint and texture, it paused, turning the corner into the bedroom. Then dug in again, louder, closer, mocking.

Night after night, I lay stiff as a board and trusted God was in control. At this point, I was fed up and ready for a fight. Releasing my wife's hand, I pounced from the bed expecting to come face-to-face with a sadistic demon, only to be met by silence. Chasing after it out into the kitchen, I flipped the light on, but still nothing. "Come out and fight. I'm tired of your games," I said, taunting and throwing my arms up, begging for a brawl. After a few minutes of silence, my fists relaxed, and my breathing slowed. "Cowards. All of you," I murmured, leaning on the kitchen island.

Looking at the microwave, I remembered I had skipped dinner, and there was a plate of food in the microwave. I grabbed a bottle of bourbon and a short glass in one hand and pulled the dish from the microwave with the other. I was going to show the evil spirits who was boss by preparing a table in front of them. I left myself wide open by walking out the back door. Setting everything down on the small patio table, I prepared my feast. "Come and get me," I growled, shutting the back door. Knowing it might be my last meal, I turned on the gas fireplace to enjoy it.

Staring into the blazing fire, I was reminded of the possessed journal hiding around the side of the house. If it was the source, it was time for a standoff. I squeezed between the propane tank and the fence in the darkness, finding it after a few blind passes of my hand. Returning to the porch, I briefly sat on the steps and gazed at the heavens. There were no stars as I gripped the journal, praying to cleanse the book and bind any spirits latched to it.

Taking my seat, I watched the flames dance through the bottle of bourbon. First, I cut the chicken into perfectly sized pieces, then savored each bite while staring at the defeated journal. Raising the bourbon-filled glass with the last swallow of the meal, I presented a toast to my fallen enemy. I swirled the glass and leaned back on the loveseat, savoring the sweet aroma inches from my tastebuds.

"What do you think you are doing?" my wife shouted, ripping the glass from my hand.

"What does it look like?" I launched back at her, nearly coming off the ground in shock.

Trying to snatch back the glass, she pulled away even further. A half bottle of bourbon free for the taking sat between her look of disgust and my need for a drink. I grabbed it by the neck and tipped it up, and before she could blink, I was already chugging.

"Stop it; put it down," she screamed, grabbing the raised bottle with her empty hand and yanking it free. The anger in her eyes flashed to fright as I lunged from my seat.

"I wanted a drink, just one. Take it, though. I don't care," I said, grabbing the empty plate and turning off the fireplace.

She would understand if she knew half of what I'd been through. She was at the kitchen sink, dumping the bourbon straight down the drain before I made it through the door after her. Her knuckles were white from clenching the sink with her free hand as she stared me down through eyes of rage. Why? I wasn't sure, but we were safe, and that's all that mattered.

CHAPTER 9

The next day I planted myself on a lounge chair, hypnotized by the waterfalls crashing into the pool below. There were three, much like the Holy Trinity. God's voice poured out before me, the sound of many waters. The bright pink flowers rested in their pots, the sun reflected on top of the water, and beautiful creations were all around.

"Honey, you need to come inside and eat. You've been out here since this morning, walking the yard barefoot. You're getting sunburnt," my wife said, putting her hand on my shoulder. "Come on, you've been out here long enough."

Shaking my shoulder and pleading couldn't move me from the presence of God. He was all around. The wind rippled through the treetops, the songbirds sung, and even a sweet burning smell floated through the air like the Holy Spirit hovering before the earth was formed.

"Well, stay out here if you want," she said, "but you have an appointment later we can't miss."

An appointment was good. It meant the plan was set into motion.

She didn't know why I had walked the yard for hours that morning, but I hoped we'd be gone before she found out. At first, the sporadic silver-dollar size holes in the yard looked like nothing more than rodent dens and uncovered squirrel pantries. Innocent enough, but as I strolled barefoot, in and around the occasional spot, they led deeper into the yard. The holes became more condensed and methodical. It was there with my feet surrounded, looking around, when I noticed the holes were running in perfect lines in every direction. I was in the middle of thousands of blast holes charged with explosives. One wrong move and everything would blow. There wouldn't be anything left of the house or the yard. It took me hours to return to the patio, one tiny, meticulous step at a time. Either someone wanted me dead or had tried to make it look like I died in a freak explosion.

Returning a few hours later, her voice was sharp and quick. "Honey, come on. We have to go."

It was go time. I kept my head down so satellite cameras couldn't catch a shot of my face. We moved quickly into and through the house. Throwing on a ball cap and deck shoes with no time to spare, we hopped into her car and backed out of the drive. As we pulled away, I glanced at our beautiful home one last time, knowing I'd never set foot inside those walls again. It would be leveled to a pile of ashes with the click of a button, removing all evidence of my existence. Leaning my head on the door as we barreled down the road, I watched the lines run between the brim of my hat and the plastic-trimmed door. I knew I would see my children again, but I wasn't sure if it would be in this life or the next.

***

The radio was set to the same Christian station, but the music broke up with patchy static. I was convinced someone was tracking us through the stereo. My wife was swerving in and out of cars like a stunt driver. Maybe she knew more about what was happening than she was letting on. Why else would she be so panicked? I trusted she would keep me safe or die trying.

Coming to a stop, I lifted my head enough to see we were stuck at a red light, surrounded on three sides by cars. From under the bill of my hat, I could see my wife fidgeting with her phone like it was on fire, but she wouldn't set it down no matter how much it burned. Beyond her, the oncoming traffic roared by us, shaking the car. These poor folks had no idea the rapture was at hand. What would they do if they knew today might be their last day? Would they still be running here and there like a bunch of scrambling ants?

Glancing right, a shiny red sedan with tinted windows pounced forward, engine revving, wanting to be noticed. The driver's window descended, revealing the side profile of a square-jawed man, face forward and rigid. His hands gripped the wheel at ten and two, rolling his fingers. With a snap of his head, we were eye to eye without his torso flinching. My window and a few feet of pavement stood between us and his hollow, soulless eyes. Before, this would have scared me, but now I felt bad for him and all the others who let evil spirits hop in and out of their bodies.

The light turned green, and our wheels shifted forward. The man gave an eerie, see-you-soon wave and chuckled. We left him behind, turning left and up an incline as I sank my head below the window again. They were going to chase us wherever we went. My heart pounded as we stopped again. It's safe not to look, but I knew we had to be boxed in. I couldn't let them make eye contact again. They might be trying to hijack my body. With my wife still shaking, phone in hand, texting, I knew we were in trouble. Whoever was on the other end must be giving her orders. I hoped she knew what she was doing.

Still not moving, I lifted my head enough to see we were in a fast food drive-through. Ducking in there was a good maneuver to throw them off our tail. Her phone dinged, and she hammered the gas, shooting us out of line. We must have sat still too long and blown our cover. We barreled down the road again, and I wouldn't look around this time. If they couldn't see my eyes, the demons giving chase wouldn't know who I was, and maybe we'd make it to wherever we were headed.

"We're going to be early," she said as the car slowed quite a bit.

We were off the highway, so I peeked over the door like a small child to see another parking lot. We were lined up against a building, another drive-through.

"I'm getting you something to eat. It's going to be a while before you get another chance," she said, pulling next to the menu.

She knew where we were headed, but why wasn't she telling me? After eating, she handed over the rest of hers as we careened down the highway again. Leaning against the window, I saw wildflowers whipping by, leaving iridescent blue, purple, and yellow trails in their wake like glowsticks at a rave.

"Look how beautiful the flowers are," I said in awe of their majesty. "So vibrant and alive."

"Those are weeds, honey," she said as we veered toward an exit ramp. "Not flowers."

Coming upon cars at a red light, I tipped the bill of my hat down again, hoping we were close to our destination. After several left and right turns, braking and speeding up, the car stopped. My heart thumped with excitement as I straightened up in the seat. We were facing a thick green hedge a few feet taller than the hood, and behind us, in the mirror, a red brick office building. It was a beautiful building, but I had no idea where we were. Sitting up taller, my hat hit the roof. On the other side of the hedge was an open field running up to a paved road a few hundred yards away.

"We're early," she said. "We'll have to sit tight for now."

Looked like we were hiding out behind some shrubs to me. The open field had plenty of room for an evac chopper to touch down. I was sure Secret Service was en route to secure the area. I bet they wanted to see if we could make the trip without getting poached before sending in the troops. The sound of helicopter blades cutting the air in the distance broke the silence. I strained for a glimpse, and a faint outline appeared, then vanished into the cloud cover. It was pointed in the wrong direction, but it could be clearing the airspace or running a diversion.

Gunshots rang out from behind the car and sent a shockwave through my body. They were here. The Secret Service had made it. Shouting short commands, they sounded like they were breaching the building. After a few seconds, the commotion dissipated. They must have gained entry. Shifting back and forth, I couldn't force myself to turn around and see the carnage or how close we came to dying ourselves. Maybe the chopper came later after a debriefing inside. Why else would they clear it out? I sank back in the seat, thankful they made it in time. Now we could enjoy the sunset while waiting for the "appointment."

With the last color draining from the sky, my wife looked at me and said, "It's time to go in now."

Entering under the cover of darkness made perfect sense for safety. As we crossed the parking lot, the glow from the glass front doors illuminated the giant brick columns towering above the entrance. At the base, in between and snaking around the columns, was an island of landscape weaved with color growing out of the cold concrete. Fresh splatter-stains soaked the pavement in front of a bench. It was hard to make out the color through the shadows, but I knew the source.

Hand in hand, my wife led us through the first set of sliding glass doors. She stopped at a pedestal holding a box of masks and a jug of hand sanitizer as they shut behind us. Handing me one, she put her own on, and we walked through the next pair of automatic doors to a receptionist counter. My wife talked to the lady behind the counter while I examined the room from a few steps back. There were way more people in here than I thought there would be, and I couldn't figure out why it wasn't empty.

Two ladies behind the counter were in scrubs, one filing papers, the other talking to my wife. Following the counter around was a set of sturdy wooden doors with a sliver of vertical glass in each. To our left was a full-on waiting room, with a television mounted at the far end.

Turning around with a clipboard in hand, my wife whispered, "Put your mask on."

Leading the way to the center row of seats, the chairs were pinned back-to-back, running the length of the room. We sat in the open seats, halfway down on the side, facing the glass wall now blacked out by the night sky. It was lined with chairs staring back at us from three feet away, and every seat was full. The television on the wall was running the news without sound. Explosions and riots; it was complete chaos. Trying to figure out what part of the world this was happening in, my ears were perked by the rumbling of whispers.

"It's him, look," the lady across from us said, nudging

her husband.

"How could he do such a thing?" whimpered another in disgust.

"That's him. That's him. That's the guy," said a man waving his phone at us.

The whispers echoed off the walls from every direction. Compounding and climbing over one another, taunting me. The lady in the first chair smirked, and her whisper became a growl, then a cackle. The heavyset man next to her followed suit. One by one, down the row, each vessel was overtaken by evil spirits bubbling to the surface to greet me. Too weak to inflict harm, these little cackling spirits were no different than the swarming crows. What a shame these people were so easily overtaken. Almost like they wanted to be controlled. No fight in them at all.

Tired of listening to their madness after a few minutes, I slipped the mask over my face and stood to stretch my legs. Walking toward the front desk, I saw two cameras mounted to the ceiling in the corner. Both were facing the same direction but were pointed at different angles. Left at the corner led to a dead end, blocked by the wooden doors. Turning back to the cameras, the angles led to a couple framed papers, one on top of the other. The bottom frame displayed a license to operate a chiropractor's office, and the top was a podiatry license. What kind of appointment were we supposed to be having here? This must be some sort of bait-and-switch scheme. Depending on which camera was pulled, they could hide whatever they wanted to.

The first opening to the right of the frames was the men's room, followed by the women's further down the wall. In the middle was a scanner mounted about four feet up the wall. I was convinced it was a retina scanner. Putting it low so ordinary people wouldn't think anything of it was genius. I pressed my face against the scanner. First, my left eye, then the right. Leaning in with a hand on either side of the small blank screen, I saw nothing. Not even a flicker. I made another pass, holding them in place longer for a better scan. Again, nothing. The screen didn't turn on, and the doors didn't fly open. I was missing the key to level up.

With that, I was off for some fresh air, bypassing the front desk, ripping the mask away, and strolling out the doors. The air was too thick in there, anyway. The crisp night air filled my lungs outside the doors as I stretched out my arms and sat on the bench. I saw so many stains on the ground, but no blood. They were good at cleaning up after themselves. The light from the foyer reached far enough to illuminate the red and yellow flowers at the base of the columns against the pitch-black night. From the bushes hovering over the flowers emerged a baby bunny. Staring into each other's eyes, it wiggled its little nose at me before hopping off. Cracking a smile, I stood to head back in and said, "I see you, Lord, and thank you. I needed that."

Breaching the doors and grabbing a new mask, I noticed the wall opposite where we sat was lined with lockers. A woman removed a bag from one of them on the bottom row. Watching in pure interest, we almost collided as she stormed by in a huff and out the doors. Maybe she failed her test, and they had sent her packing. The receptionists were still working away. So much so they didn't notice the hands on the clock above their heads were spinning backward. Plopping down next to my wife, I leaned into her shoulder, trying to avoid eye contact with everyone.

"Hi, James. How are you?" rang out from above.

"Oh, hey. I'm fine. Glad you're here," I said. It was my

mother-in-law in her work scrubs and shiny nurse shoes.

She sat beside my wife, and I settled back in. Avoiding eye contact didn't help. The spirits could smell me and began welling up from the depths of the vessels lining the wall. Whispers and growls seeped from the curled lips and gnashing teeth encircling us. Jumping up again, I bolted for the bathroom. It was just a matter of time before one of those spirits got brave enough to attack, and I shouldn't be next to my wife when it happened. Locking the door behind me and ripping the mask off, I leaned over the sink to rinse my face in cold water. I told myself I was strong enough to handle it.

I left the bathroom after a few minutes and tried the scanner again. Leaning in, I shifted left, then right, but nothing. Circular motion up close and then further out, but still nothing. Not a single beep or flash. I had to go back outside and start at the beginning again because I wasn't doing something right. Glancing at the clock behind the counter as I headed for the door, it was now at a standstill, but I didn't have time to figure it out. I bolted through the glass sliders to the bench and laid down this time, feet up and hands tucked behind my head. Cold metal bars dug into my back, but it was quieter than inside. Soft footsteps marched up the pavement from a distance, growing heavier the closer they got, like a marching soldier.

"Yes, sir. He's way better than the others. He's already lasted longer than any of them. Keep it going? Yes, sir," said a firm voice from a few yards away.

Rolling to see who was speaking, the voice matched the person. A dark T-shirt tucked with precision into pressed khaki pants and black boots shined so much the stars could see their reflection. He saw me staring, dropped his hand, turned, and marched into the darkness. It was a test, and I was right. Setting my feet on the ground, I had to get back inside and keep this thing moving. Grabbing another mask on the way in, I planted myself next to my wife again. She was clueless.

The whispers crept in again like fog rising in a swamp. Inaudible murmurs crawled around the room, tugging at our feet, trying to pull us into the depths with them. From behind, a childish giggle piggybacked the whispering. It grew louder and louder until the sadistic laughter bellowed off the walls. I jumped to my feet, and it became silent. Nothing but smoke and mirrors, vanishing before I could turn and fight. Since I was up, I went outside again, hoping it would follow me.

This time, bypassing the bench, I ventured out to the flowerbed island at the feet of the columns. Leaning down and picking each vibrant flower to smell, I worked around the circle and back to where the first flower fell from my fingers. The tiny rabbit was gone. Maybe he made it through the hedge into the wide-open field. Walking around the middle of the parking lot, I stared into the field until a somber cry from the sidewalk broke my focus. A man drowning in sorrow sat hunched in the shadows over the curb and swaying. Hairs on my neck shot up, and chills electrified my skin. The sobs weren't natural. Watching with reluctant curiosity, he rocked to a slow stop, head still buried in tightly crossed arms. Sobs slowed to whimpers, then to silence. His mangled hair hadn't been washed in months, and the torn shirt falling from his shoulders hadn't been either.

His face flashed upward, staring back, lip quivering. "Hey!" he shouted, springing from the pavement. "Come here, boy," he growled, motioning with his decrepit hand.

He was about the same distance from me as I was to

the entrance. If I ignored him and didn't show fear, maybe he'd leave me alone. I spun toward the doors as his taunts got louder. Halfway to the glass sliders, his feet broke loose from the pavement. Screaming jumbled up profanity, he was barreling down on me. I bolted through the entrance, he was so close my neck was burning from his breath. We burst through the foyer, and he stopped the pursuit, belting an earsplitting scream. It continued until I reached my seat, trembling. Latching onto my wife, I looked up for the first time to see his body rocking back and forth. He was head down and shaking with violent sobs as slobber pooled around his worn and dirty bare feet.

Again, the faint whispers rolled through the room, like evil spirits climbing from one chair to the next, filling the room with painful moans and terrified weeping as more joined in. In unison, the room merged into one rhythmic symphony of pain and chaos, echoing like the spirits of an ancient dungeon. Adrenaline welled up inside me, with nowhere to go. The doorway was blocked, and there was nowhere to go but deeper.

"Mr. Coast, you can come back now," said a smiling woman in scrubs with a clipboard.

CHAPTER 10

We followed the nurse around the corner to where she stopped. Pulling an ID card from her waist, she pressed it against the waist-high retina scanner. The fortified doors swung open with a beep, revealing a long, dark hallway. Light escaped from the small windows carved in the doors on either side, illuminating small sections of our path. Framed pictures of wildlife and nature scenes devoid of color filled the space between each open doorway. Our footsteps bounced through the empty hall as she showed us to our room. Stark-white and barren walls encased the private cube. A few plastic chairs and a boxed-in television hanging from the corner greeted us upon entering.

"Someone will be with you shortly," the nurse said, shutting the door behind her.

Trying to figure out why the antique television was hanging from the wall encased in plexiglass, I panicked, thinking the door might have locked behind us.

Snapping to my feet and grabbing the door, my wife asked, "What are you doing? Leave the door alone." But it was already open, and I was already peering into the dim hallway. Not a soul in either direction, and a few steps into the darkness, not a sound to be heard. To the right, at the end of the hall, were the doors we came in through. Little slivers of light bled in from the lobby. To the left, a pair of the same-style doors guarded the hallway, but no glimmer of light came from them.

They drew me in as I passed a third set of doors, enthralled by what hid behind them. A new level? My next test? How much longer was this going to take? It was too dark beyond the doors to see anything through the glass. Tapping the wooden frame and looking for a way to open them, I thought the small map mounted next to them might be the key. Leaning over and studying the maze of hallways and doors proved useless. The map couldn't have been accurate. The halls ran in circles around the center of the building, broken up by countless doors. Some that led to nowhere. I was on my own to figure this maze out and still at square one.

A frame down the hall cast a faint glow as the light poured from our room, kissing the wall beside it. I walked back toward it thinking it must be a clue. Lots of framed pictures lined the walls, but that one was illuminated. With my hands behind my back, I inspected the frame and its contents. A field full of beautiful wildflowers, majestic mountains in the background, and a handful of trees stood firm. Searching into the depths of the picture produced nothing.

Strolling back into the lit room, the conversation between my wife and mother-in-law halted as I crossed the threshold.

"The picture out there is amazing," I said, scooting the last empty chair from the wall so I could put my feet up. Maybe I could coax them into checking the picture out themselves. After a few minutes of baiting, nothing worked, and they didn't budge. Since they weren't helping me find clues, I had more exploring to do on my own.

This time I went back the way we came in. Light from the windows guided me like hope in the darkness. Halfway down the hall, I saw a man through the narrow window. He was staring at me, cell phone in hand, leaning back in a chair. His foot was propped up by a teal blue suitcase, rolling back and forth. I knew he must be waiting out there for me. Looking over my shoulder, I bolted to the doors, waving to get his attention. It was too dark in the hall; he couldn't see me. Yanking on the door handles did nothing. I was trapped. Banging on the doors would bring unwanted attention.

After another round of dissecting the painting for clues, I returned to the sterile room. My wife was in there, and I knew she was safe in the light. Frustration grew with these games, though, and I was ready to get beyond the amateur tests and holding tanks. Not more than a few minutes sitting, and I needed out again. The whitewashed walls were surgical, and the room was cold. If the door locked, we were done for. No way out.

One more inspection of the field on the wall produced nothing. Disappointed, I paced the hall toward the doors with the blacked-out windows. It looked like a set of doors on the surface. Their purpose was more like a dam, but what were they holding back? Before I got halfway, light beaming from a door pulled me to the left. Through the narrow glass sat two young girls against the back wall. The frizzy-haired blonde had her feet pulled up on the chair and her head buried in her knees. The much smaller girl was draped over her in tears and must have been the younger sister. Both were trembling with fear, trapped, and all alone. Nothing I could do to help, but if I found a way out, I'd come back for them.

Turning back to the doors, I carried on to the end of the looming hallway. I had to find out what they were holding back. Placing my palm where the two doors met, they began to shake within seconds. Loud cracks of someone trying to kick it down, again and again, threw me off-balance. The vibration died, and the beating stopped. From between the doors, gentle whispers floated out. Leaning in to make them out, my ear hovered inches from the wood, but silence. A deafening silence draped the doorway but was soon ripped away.

"We're waiting for you," whispered a decrepit female voice.

"Come join us," cackled a drove of growling followers.

"Yes, come join us."

Jumping back from the door, my back slammed against the wall. *Go toward the light,* I told myself, gathering my composure before returning to the room.

Waiting continued for hours on end with nothing to do but stare at the surgically sterile room. The sound of a door latching carried down the hall to our room, accompanied by the echo of a shaky metal cart being drug across the tiles. From the darkness emerged a nurse pushing a small screen on a metal stick with wheels.

"The intake specialist will be with you in a few minutes," she said, fading into the shadows of the hallway.

All three of us were now awake and alert, sitting at attention. Waiting patiently for the screen to come alive. Odd approach, but top-secret government missions couldn't be taken lightly, I supposed.

In the silence, it dawned on me why the people from the first waiting room scoffed and looked at their phones. It must have been my house. The charges must have been blown, and I was being framed for it. With all those holes in the yard, there wouldn't be anything left. I was walking around the yard, and someone must have recorded me. I didn't do it, though. They couldn't lock me up for something I didn't do. My wife wouldn't do that to me. This must be a test, a vetting process to see if I could keep my cool. I had seen movies about these kinds of mind games.

After a few moments, the screen powered on and displayed static. The static soon gave way to a lady enshrouded in red, rattling like a tambourine as her bracelets hit the table before her. Large wooden beads the size of golf balls wrapped around her neck. She smiled and ran through the usual introduction pleasantries with my wife. Her eyes were as red as the wrap towering over her head. She had all the makings of a real live witch doctor. Brought all the way from who knows where, straight to my room. She wasn't getting a straight answer out of me. I let my wife handle the questions. She couldn't see past the façade, but they wouldn't get to her.

"Sir, hi there," the woman in red said. "How many children do you have?"

"Kids, none," I said. Even if I did, she'd be the last to know.

"So, you don't have any children at home?"

Shaking my head, I said, "I think I would know if I did."

After some back and forth, she turned her eyes to my wife and said I should be admitted for observation, which might take up to a week. Relief flooded my body because my wife and mother-in-law could leave and get to safety. The screen went dim, and I pushed it to the side. My eyes welled up with tears when my wife put her hand on my back.

"It's going to be okay, honey," she said. "I promise."

As she rubbed my back, I couldn't help but think how sad she looked at the thought of leaving me behind.

"They might offer you medicine, but you don't have to take anything you don't want to," said my mother-in-law leaning forward. "You can ask, and they have to tell you what it is and what it's supposed to do, but they can't force you to take anything."

"Okay, good," I responded.

At that point, it made sense why she was there. As a nurse, she was there to deliver those words of wisdom. Heeding her words, I didn't plan on taking anything, and they would have had to hold me down to make me.

"What are you doing?" I asked my wife as she pulled the laces from my shoes.

"You can't have these while you're in here," she said.

I wondered if they thought I was an escape artist. What would I have used those for anyway? The thuds of much larger shoes made their way to our door. A man in scrubs, much larger than myself, hovered in the doorway. He motioned for me to follow as my wife leaned in for a fierce embrace. Letting go, my mother-in-law also reached for a hug, and I followed the man into the darkness. We walked to the left, toward the end of the hall where the spirits hid beyond the doors, waiting.

With a scan of his ID, the lock popped free, and he pushed through the doors like they were made of paper. We entered another dim, rectangular room as the doors latched behind us. It was a common area lined with open doors up and down the far wall. Void of life. The depth of darkness seeping from the doorways held the room. I was but a guest. A faint glow rose from several computers behind the U-shaped counter to my right. "Follow me," he said, noticing me lag behind.

He weaved between the chairs of a small seating area with a short cube in the center for a table. Following on his heels, it almost took me out as his broad shoulders blocked what little light there was.

Following the glow to the far side, he pulled out a chair from underneath a cutout in the counter. Motioning for me to sit, he walked off the way we came, fading into the room. To my left, the same faint computer glow projected from a small sliding glass window in the wall.

"Fill these out for me," commanded a female's voice, sliding her chair into view.

She dropped a small stack of papers and a pencil nub on the counter. Plopping onto the seat, I grabbed the nub and laid my head against the wall, scribbling on the top page. Ripping the paper from underneath my hand, she slammed it back down.

"Sign here," she said, pointing to a line on the page.

After working through the stack, she set them aside.

"This is your water cup," she said, slamming a clear plastic cup with a straw in front of me. "You can refill it at the machines on either end of the room. Now stick out your arm." Grabbing my hand, she flipped it upside down and wrapped a paper bracelet around my wrist. "We're ready," she called out over her shoulder.

The man who escorted me reappeared from the shadows and motioned for me to follow. Not moving from my seat, he walked the entire length of the counter to get me. Before he reached arm's length, I stood and snatched the cup. Following him back the way we came, he stopped at what looked like a closet door between where we entered and the half-moon desk. Fishing in his pocket, he pulled out a set of keys and narrowed them down to the one that unlocked the door. As the key twisted in the knob, the lady from behind the desk walked up behind us and followed us in. It was a cramped laundry room. As I was looking at the racks of baskets and shelves of towels, the door locked behind us.

"Take off your shoes," said the man sliding the keys back into his pocket.

"Now take your shirt off and drop your shorts."

"Facing us, open the waistband of your underwear."

"Now turn in a circle."

"Good, you can put your clothes and shoes back on now. The items you'll need for daily hygiene are on this rack in front of you. They stay locked up in here, and you need to ask for assistance. Someone will get them for you."

With that, he opened the door, and the lady led me

through the darkness to a door on the far wall. "This one's yours," she said, flipping the light switch and walking off.

Two steps in, on the left, was a bathroom with a poor excuse for a door. It was a swinging saloon door offering zero chance of privacy. A set of twin beds laid out beneath barren walls filled the rest of the room, except for some shelves mounted at the foot of the beds. I wondered who the second bed was for as I opened the window blinds. They revealed a small courtyard encased in a towering wrought-iron fence. I ran my fingers up the window frame, but there wasn't a way to open it. Collapsing backward on the bed, tears of pain and confusion poured from within. I was confused about how I got there and what I had done to deserve being put in a cage.

Wrapping myself with the one thin blanket, I stared at the wall until I regained my composure. Everything happens for a reason, even if I didn't know why. It was time to go find that reason. Peering from the doorway, the glowing window and counter were straight ahead beyond a small seating area. The lady at the counter looked busy, so I snuck out. Quickly and quietly, I moved to one of the chairs surrounding a small coffee table and sat with my back to the counter, inspecting the room. Straight ahead was a television mounted high on the wall, butted against the ceiling. To the right, my door, plus one more. Down the wall to the left was a hallway that ran beside the wall of open doors and disappeared around the corner.

Flashes of lightning lit up the ceiling through a massive skylight above my head. A thunderous storm flared as rain pounded the glass like war drums and thunder clapped. I was mesmerized by the raging beauty. God was on the warpath. This could only mean one thing: the rapture was at hand. The world was burning down outside these walls. Chaos and panic reigned as lightning burned down entire cities and waters flooded the streets. That's why this place was fortified. I was one of the chosen people to ride out the wrath of God from inside the walls.

Staring into the storm, lightning tormented the night sky, and I felt energy building within. My sins were burning from the inside out, cleansing my soul. My teeth were clenched, my fists balled up, and the center of my body was stretched toward the ceiling. The hand of God was lifting me toward the heavens. Writhing about, the force was too much for my body to handle as smoke rose from my feet.

The smell of burning skin kissed the air as I struggled to find the chair below me. An earthshaking clap of thunder released me from the air, slamming me to the seat. Smoke rose from my shoes as I yanked my singed feet from the charred socks. My feet were still intact.

The sound of soft footsteps along the wall caught my attention. One of the keepers was shining a flashlight in each room as she walked past the open doorways. I deduced she was doing a head count to see who had already been taken in the rapture and who was still left. Walking closer, she blinded me with the light when she noticed my curiosity. She hit me a second time when I tried to reopen them. With my hand up in retreat, my face was to the floor until the footsteps were out of range.

Now behind the counter with the other lady, they whispered back and forth. It was time to explore a little. I followed the wall under the television to the hallway and disappeared around the corner, throwing my socks in the trash can along the way. The poorly lit hallway revealed twenty more feet of doors running down the left side, dying into a wall with a glass door at its center. To my right, a fountain drink machine sat perched on the counter next to a refrigerator. Walking toward the doors, beyond the counter hung one lone shelf. On it were various books for coloring and reading, as well as puzzles.

I dug through the pile and uncovered a small King James Bible. Bible in hand, I inspected the locked door. It led to another small room, a foyer, with the outside world beyond it. A fluorescent green circle mounted on the exterior wall cut through the darkness. Mantis also controlled this facility, but how was I supposed to get out? Shaking the door and looking for levers or buttons to push, it was apparent this wasn't the way. At least not yet. Maybe something else came first.

The same fluorescent green beckoned from the opposite side of the room. Not wanting to pass near the open doors, I cut through the seating area and hugged the counter, stopping in the center of the room. The arch of the counter spanned from one wall to within feet of the opposite wall. I was splitting a doorway that would separate the space into identical halves if it were shut.

"What are you doing, Mr. James?" asked one of the ladies behind the counter.

"Nothing. Going to sit down over there and read is all."

Moving through the doorway, I picked a seat facing the counter, not trusting them at my back. The Bible flipped open to the book of James, and my eyes strained to work through the words in low light. My arm peeled from the stiff, pleather armchair with every page turn. I was striving to focus, but the ladies behind the counter proved to be better entertainment. Whispering back and forth, followed by short bursts of laughter, like schoolgirls in a library. From this angle, they wore matching scrubs. They could have been nurses, but I wasn't sure.

Without warning, the air erupted with a bang from the wooden doors bursting behind me. They got another one. She must have made it into the building before the rapture. Head sunk low, walking behind the gatekeeper, she may have been better off outside. The shadow of her ballcap hid her face, but her short, narrow frame suggested she was late teens or early twenties. Stopping at the laundry room door and fumbling through keys, he motioned for one of the nurses to join him, and they disappeared behind the closet door. When they reemerged, the young woman followed the nurse to the counter, jacket in hand. The man shot me a perverse grin as he disappeared through the doors.

Stooped over, weeping in the chair at the counter, the young lady shielded her eyes with one hand and clutched her jacket with the other. The nurse shoved a stack of papers in front of her, slammed the pencil nub on the counter, and told her to complete everything. Flinching, the weeping intensified with the crack of the pencil. The nurse leaned in with a scrunched nose and tightened lips glowing from the computer light.

"I said, fill these out. What's the matter with you? Don't speak English?" Weeping became sobbing. Turning to her counterpart and throwing her hands in the air, the nurse shouted, "Can you believe this? Why do I always have to deal with these ones? I don't get paid enough for this."

Turning back to the young lady, she spoke like she was dealing with a toddler. Reaching my tolerance level, I slammed the Bible on the coffee table and made it a point to jump from my seat. The shock was enough to stop the beratement. Our eyes were locked, and I watched the anger drain from her face.

"Are you done yet?" I asked, leaning over the counter toward her.

She rolled back in her chair with a blank stare but didn't say a word, so I turned my attention to the young lady. I could see the pain magnified in her eyes by the tears.

"It's going to be okay. You can come to sit by me."

Wiping her eyes on her shirt sleeve, the tears stopped flowing. By the blank look on her face, I don't think she understood my words, but the peace in my eyes brought her comfort.

Returning to my seat, she stayed in the chair, watching my every move. She looked to the nurse, then back toward me as I motioned her to the chair next to me. Wiping her face again, she sat beside me, divided by a small end table. She continued to stare with a look of pure shock on her face. Inspecting her feet and legs, she lifted her letterman jacket from her torso, then held her arms out as if it were the first time she had seen them.

"I died yesterday in a ditch along a road," she said, setting her jacket back down. "It was flooding, and I drowned. How is this possible? Did you do this?"

"No, of course not. I just got here myself. All your answers are in this little book right here, though," I said, shaking the Bible in my hand. "My God can do anything.

You must have a great calling for your life, so He brought you back."

"Please, tell me about this God of yours," she said, leaning over the side of the chair.

"What would you like me to read about? This book covers everything."

"Read me whatever you like. I want to hear it all," she said, laying her head on the arm of the chair like a child.

"I'm James by the way."

"I'm Nia."

A few pages into the book of Luke, the second nurse walked up to us and politely asked if she would like to see her room. She popped her head up and looked at the nurse, then back to me, about to panic.

"It's okay. I'm right here. I'll be sitting here all night. You'll be safe, promise," I said, motioning for her to follow. Their outlines disappeared around the corner, and I continued reading Luke.

Now in silence with the nurses behind the counter again, it seemed all was safe and sound. Finding the way back to my room, I almost lost hope. Running out of options and patience, the second-to-last door in the room had my name handwritten on a strip of paper by the door. Maybe there were some clues about what was happening in the paperwork they gave me. The red folder and half a pencil they had given me earlier that night were on the small table by the bed. The stiff bed crackled under my weight as I pulled the papers out of the folder. Words littered the front and back of all the pages. Turning them every which way produced nothing. They weren't legible. The words were all jumbled up like a code of sorts. Maybe the pencil nub was for deciphering the chaos, but I wasn't quite there yet, so I returned the papers to the folder.

Lying down with hands folded and staring at the ceiling, I wondered what the future held. *Would the sun ever come out again? Are the stars gone forever? Why were we chosen over everyone else in the world to be here? Did my wife get taken in the rapture? If not, what broken world is left out there for her?* Tears streamed from my eyes and rolled off the pillowcase as loneliness crept in to accompany me.

CHAPTER 11

As daylight broke through the window, shuffling feet and rustling plastic snuck into the room to greet me with the pleasant aroma of coffee close behind. Through the doorway, I watched a male worker put the lid on the coffee dispenser across the room. Pulling the plastic cover from the last stack of Styrofoam cups, he tossed it in the trash and disappeared through the main doors.

From my doorway, the waking sunlight fell from the skylights, bringing the common area to life. Seeing the sun again was beautiful, but it didn't do the common area any favors. Plastic armchairs in soft pastel colors formed mirror-image sitting areas on either side of the room. With its redwood counter, the nurses' station rolled through the space between them. It looked like a half-circle observation deck in the sunlight, the kind from the zoo. The long wall of doors on the right was broken up by two-person tables staggered between the openings and a handful of framed landscape pictures. If a doctor's office threw up after eating Easter candy, this would be the result.

The first one to the coffee, I sat at one of the tables along the wall and waited to see what happened next. One by one, men and women filed out of their rooms. Most went for coffee, then filled the group seating areas on both sides of the room. They all looked normal from afar, half-awake, sporting messy hair and wrinkled clothes.

In mid-sip of coffee, my line of sight was blocked by a large woman emerging from the doorway in front of my table.

Arms stretched and yawning, she turned to face me. "I thought someone was outside my door," she said, hobbling to sit across from me. "You must be new. I'm Marge. I run this place. Well, not run, but I watch out for everyone."

She got situated in her seat and pushed her round, bottle-thick glasses back into place.

"Good morning. Nice to meet you, Marge. No coffee for you?"

"No, can't have it. Gives me the shakes," she said with a laugh and twitched her fingers.

She twisted in her chair to look over her shoulder at the group seating and said, "Sorry, Jen, I didn't mean to jump in your head again."

"It's okay. Too early to barge in on anything good. Don't worry about it," a brown-haired lady from the group replied. She waved it off without even looking in our direction.

Before I could ask, Marge chuckled and said, "I can head hop. You know, read people's minds. Sometimes I can control it, and other times I can't." She shrugged her shoulders and folded her arms across her midriff. Leaning back in her chair, she asked, "What brings you here in the middle of the night? Must have been something serious."

I searched for an answer that should have been easy to find while Marge's eyes narrowed with concentration. I couldn't remember why I was there and wasn't sure what to say. She leaned in with great intent as if I was already speaking. Nervous, I broke the silence with the truth.

"I don't know. I can't remember why I'm here."

Her eyes widened as she leaned back again, adjusting

her glasses, and smiled. "Don't worry. I can't read your mind. Either that, or nothing's going on up there," she said, finishing with a belly laugh while tapping the side of her head.

Pushing herself up with the help of the table and the back of her chair, she worked to unsteady feet before letting go. "Gotta get my cigarettes," she said, letting go of the chair. "Smoke break is the only time we get to go outside."

While we were talking, a line had formed at the window in the wall for cigarette handouts. I watched a second line form at the door I had investigated last night. As the last few people collected their smokes from the window and joined the group, one of the workers pushed through to the front of the line, followed by a second.

I was scared of what may be waiting on the other side of the door, but being alone inside might be worse. Besides, nobody knew that the rapture had happened last night, and they may need my help to calm everyone down. The worker bringing up the back end ushered me in front of him as the line crawled out the door. A spacious concrete patio with a roof was waiting on the other side of the glass door.

Brick columns supported the metal roof and were connected by a bench no one sat on. Everyone had wandered off to the right, where a concrete sidewalk meandered through the bright green grass. It passed through the middle of the courtyard, bordered by benches and perfectly manicured flowerbeds. The sidewalk continued for the entire length of the enclosure and dead-ended into a uniformed worker with his arms crossed. Behind him was a gate in the towering wrought-iron fence that led to an open field spanning as far as I could see. At least a few birds had survived the night and were playing in the bushes outside the bars.

Five or six small, segregated groups huddled throughout the caged area, running the length of the building. Smoking and talking, unaware their families may have been wiped from the earth. Everyone here belonged to a group, except one older gentleman in the corner. Taking deep drags, the tails of smoke streamed from his cigarette, matching his hair in length and color as he stared at the pavement. Following the curved path, *Leave the ninety-nine for the one* echoed in my head. As I worked toward the lone man, heads turned, and whispers flared, but now was no time for distractions.

"Do you mind if I sit down?" I asked, hovering over the empty side of the bench.

"Free country last time I checked," he said, flicking the butt of his cigarette.

Taking a seat and crossing my foot over my knee, I stared off into the field for a few minutes. Trying to think of the right words to say.

"It's a beautiful day the Lord has made, isn't it?" I asked, breaking the silence.

Sparking a match, his already wrinkled face looked more like a melting candle as he puckered to light his next cigarette. He tossed the spent match, looked over, and said, "We're all going to hell anyway, so what does it matter?"

His eyes didn't appear nearly as old as the rest of his body. Thin and frail, half his wrinkles may have been loose skin from not eating, judging by the knobby spine protruding from his shirt.

"That sounds a little extreme, don't you think?"

He scoffed and ashed his cigarette on the petals of an innocent flower beside the bench. "I was a preacher for many years. Had my own church even. Humans are the evilest, vile creatures on the planet. You have no idea what I've seen with my own eyes and the stories people have told me trying to unload their sins. God is coming back with a vengeance soon, and when He does, the whole world will burn in the fiery pit of hell. If I had it my way, I'd kill them all and save God the trouble."

"Well, it sounds like you have the Old Testament wrath and damnation down, but what about the forgiveness part and love your neighbor? Isn't God the only one who can judge?"

"The Old Testament is all I ever preached from. It's the law. Without it, there's no order, and, well, look at America now. People don't want to hear the truth, that's why I quit preaching."

The anger in his voice sounded more like years of pain coming through in the only thing he'd ever known: religion. He was trapped, and his crystal-blue eyes screamed for help from behind his harsh words. The spirit of religion had him caged and singing like a tone-deaf songbird. No doubt this man had led more people away from God than to Him.

"Do you believe in Jesus?" I asked softly.

"What kind of question is that? I was a preacher; of course, I do."

"The Bible has three parts; you're missing the other two. The Old Testament is the law set by God, and Jesus came to earth as the action, or living Word, if you will. The New Testament didn't do away with the Old but became the new covenant between God and us. Father, Son, and Holy Ghost. We need all three."

Waiting for his response, nothing came but a blank stare into space. "I'll leave you with one last thing, then I'll quit bothering you. You said you believe in Jesus, and I believe you do. Since you believe in Jesus, you must believe in his works, also. All of which were among sinners like us, tax collectors, and prostitutes. Every day he was in a battle with the religious leaders of that time who were trying to enforce what they thought was the law. His disciples were all men like you and me who laid down their old ways and followed Jesus. They were far from perfect, and so are we. Sometimes religion does more harm than good, sir. You and I still need to save the ones that are left. If not us, then who?"

I rose from the cold metal bench as the groups dispersed toward the door, and I filtered in with the crowd. Piling through the door, most handed their cigarette packs in at the window. The rest disappeared to their rooms or sat around the common areas. With my back to the wall, I took up a two-seat table again and tried to read the room. Fear was so thick in the air that it was hard to see the pain and sorrow beneath the surface. Each person was made in the perfect image of God yet imprisoned by an imperfect body. Trying to claw their way out, they were bound by emotions and chained to the shadows of their infirmities.

"Hey, come join us," rang out a voice from the middle of the common area.

"Yeah, you, come on," said another lady, waving at me from a chair in the center.

The voice belonged to a peppy woman in her mid-twenties. Her pink-tipped, frizzy blonde curls bounced as she waved me over. Joining the small group, I took the empty spot on the floor next to her. A few others sat on the floor also, gathered around the mint green, cube-shaped coffee table. Some were coloring torn-out pages from complex and intricate coloring books, while others were scribbling over the lines on grade school cartoon characters.

"Grab a picture and start coloring," she said with wide eyes glowing through her tinted hippy glasses. "Come on. It's relaxing."

Judging by her shaky hands and quickened speech, I wasn't sure if it was, but I joined in. Grabbing the first book on top and flipping it to an unmarked page toward the back, I laid it on the table. Next to the open page on the table was a perfect row of crayons. It ran from the darkest green to the lightest, followed by the yellows. Grabbing a green from the center, no sooner than it met the paper, a shriek rang over my shoulder, and a coloring book crashed to the floor.

Jumping to my feet in shock, my newfound friend was rocking back and forth, wailing and picking at her spring-like curls.

With a gentle tug on my shirt, a sweet old lady said, "Those are her crayons, honey. Never touch her crayons. Hi, you can call me 'Ma.'"

"Hi," I said, shaking her outstretched hand.

"She'll be good in a couple of hours, happens every day. Let's go line up for breakfast, hun. I never let the new people eat alone."

I followed her to the line forming at the entry doors, where the gatekeeper ushered in new residents. Ma was the only one who looked showered and ready for the day. I remember thinking she must have worked there, because it would have explained her kind demeanor and put-together appearance.

Moments later, we were led through the doors in a single-file line. Our shoes squeaked and echoed as we entered an empty, whitewashed hall. One worker led the way, a second paced the length of the line, and a third followed from behind. When we came to an abrupt halt, I leaned over Ma's shoulder and asked why.

Raising her hand as if to push an imaginary button, she paused. The clank of doors latching behind us rippled through the hallway.

"They make sure we're locked in here like cattle before they open the next door," she said, pulling her frayed, salt-and-pepper hair into a ponytail.

The line moved forward again, turning through the sole open door carved in the endless hallway. Hugging the wall, we weaved through the cafeteria serving line. Ma led the way past row after row of picnic table seating to the center of the room.

"I like to see the whole room," she said, leaning toward me. "There are some real weirdos in here. Word to the wise: if you're in the center, you have more directions to run."

A small group filled in around us. A young adult couple sat across from us. They couldn't have been over eighteen, but their eyes suggested they were in love, nonetheless. Nia, from last night, sat in the corner alone, still wearing the ball cap. I thought about what Ma said, and she was right: no one should eat alone. "I'll be right back," I said, hiking my legs out from under the table.

From underneath the bill of her hat, she didn't see me walking toward her. Not until my third try at "Hello" did she look up.

"Come sit with us," I said. "You shouldn't be alone." Nothing but a blank stare in return, but it wasn't enough to give up. "Please, we'd like you to join us so you're not alone."

Turning toward Ma and the others, they all motioned for her to come to sit, but she remained motionless.

"We'll be right over there if you change your mind,"

I said, walking off.

I didn't think I got through and wondered if she understood me. She didn't look afraid to talk—more like she didn't understand. Seconds after I took my seat, she brought her tray and sat next to the young couple as they welcomed her.

"Why are you here?" asked Ma, tilting her head toward me. "No secrets among friends."

"I don't remember why. I just remember being here. I was in a room, with my wife and mother-in-law."

"That's intake. You don't remember why they brought you?" she asked.

I searched for answers but hit an unpassable wall. Whispers and giggles from up and down the table crept in and choked out my struggling attempt to find those memories. Staring at the untouched plate of food in front of me, tears spilled to the surface.

"It's okay," said Ma patting my back. "You'll remember soon enough. It'll come back to you. Try and eat something."

Pushing the food around on the plate the rest of the time, relief came when one of the workers announced it was time for everyone to clean up and get in line. Food went in the trash, and trays went on the metal rack. Single-file line again, we were ushered back the way we came. I hurried to my room, hoping to find clues and unlock memories.

Nothing. The shelves were bare, and no clothes were hanging from the empty wooden rods. The bathroom was also barren. There wasn't a single familiar thing. The paper tag on the wall beside the door and this paper bracelet were the only remnants of who I was. What if my name wasn't even James? Sitting on the bed, I ripped the bracelet from my wrist and threw it to the floor. The folder on the end table was the only item in the room not bolted down. The words on the pages still didn't make sense.

"Hiya!" rang out from the doorway behind me.

To my surprise, a bubbly little spirit was hopping at my door. Her hair almost touched the ground and her crossed eyes were magnified by clear-framed glasses. Her smile jumped from ear to ear.

"Whatcha doin' in there? Come on out. Please, please, please. Come on. I can't come and get you. You have to come out on your own."

Folder in hand, I wondered why this character wanted me out of the room. Maybe I would find some answers. Meeting her at the edge of the doorway, she backed up enough to let me squeeze through.

"What now?" I asked, shifting the folder to my other hand.

"Where's your bracelet?" she asked, holding her hands against her face like I was about to be in trouble.

"I don't have one."

"Oh goody, goody, goody. That's what I thought," she said, clapping her hands and jumping like a bouncy ball.

"What does that mean?" I asked, now wondering if I'd made a mistake.

"Sometimes they send guys like you that they're trying to hide for a while," she said, leaning in like it was a secret. "Didn't you see all the cameras? They put you in here to have proof you weren't out there. Most of the time, it's because someone is trying to frame you for something big. Either that or you're famous, and you don't want us to know who you are. I'm Sarah, by the way, but you can call me 'Squeaks.'"

"My house, the explosion. I remember the explosion."

"Ohhhh, I knew it! Come with me, I know what to do."

With nothing to lose, I followed her to the glass door from this morning's smoke break.

"Okay, look around. No cameras, right? Hold the folder tight like you mean business. We're going to walk straight to the door at the other end of the hall. Keep your chin up and look around like you're inspecting the room. Got it?"

I was confused, but maybe she knew what she was doing. She skipped out in front, pointing at the chairs, the floor, and the nurse's desk. Motioning with her chin to lift mine as we passed the fountain drink machine, toured the common areas, and entered the short hall at the opposite end. Coming to the door, she paused, leaned over, and laughed as she turned around.

"That was kinda okay, but no one is going to believe your performance. We need to do it again. This time, act like you mean it."

"Mean what?" I asked, frustrated with her laughter.

"Ughhhh, men are so stupid," she said, smacking her forehead. "The cameras, doofus. We need to make it look like you're here to inspect the place like you want to buy it. You don't want people to think you were locked in a looney bin, do you? Imagine if that hit the news. Now your handlers can pull the recordings and make it look like you were taking a tour."

Walking by me to peer around the corner, she motioned for me to come closer. "Ready?" she asked, looking back. "Annnnd, action." She bounced into the open with a twirl.

Walking with my chest puffed out and chin up a few feet behind her, I tried my best. After all, what if she was right about me being a visitor? She twirled the length of the room a second time. Looking like a half-wound, antique jewelry box, she jerked to a stop and lost balance each time she pointed and pretended to talk.

Reaching the other side, she turned and patted me on the shoulder. "You did good, kid. Real good." Bouncing away, she laughed and said, "Have your people call my people."

As she hopped around the corner, a head popped out of the doorway before me to see her off as well. Strawberry hair as thick and stiff as straw dangled from the end of a pale white neck supported by frog-like fingers gripping the door frame. "Finally! She's too much for me," she said, stepping forward and turning in my direction. "You want to see my paintings?"

"Sure," I replied, following her neon orange shirt into the room. Her hair shifted, revealing a glowing yellow cross in the middle of her back. She took me to the first twin bed, where two coloring book pictures lay on the covers.

Grabbing one in each hand, she lifted them up. "See? They're not really paintings, though. Those are at home. I have my own studio. This is all I had to work with."

"They're still beautiful," I said with a smile.

I turned to leave, but she grabbed my arm and spun me around. Flipping one of the pictures over, shaking it wildly, she pointed at the bottom. "What do you see?" she asked.

"It looks like a phone number."

"It's mine," she said, digging under the blanket with her free hand. She pulled out a cordless phone and shook both in my face. "The phones don't work. I need help. I was in the car with my husband, and the next thing I know, I woke up here."

"Same with me. My wife left me here last night. Let me see the phone. I'll give it a try."

Phone in hand, I strained to see the numbers to dial. "Hurry," she said. "We're not supposed to have phones in our rooms."

Holding the phone to my ear, a dial tone shouted back. Of course, the rapture took out the phones. Her husband must have been taken up right after he dropped her off. Not having the heart to tell her, I pretended to dial again. I wasn't going to be the one to break the news.

"Sorry, I didn't get through. Maybe try again in a little while?"

Handing her the phone, she erupted in tears and collapsed to her knees as I inched backward toward the door. Before she could look up, I backed out of the room and was about to turn when something caught my feet and almost sent me flying.

"Whatcha doin' in there?" asked Squeaks. "You're not supposed to be in someone else's room."

"She wanted to show me some pictures she made. That's all."

Tilting sideways to peer around me briefly, she

straightened back up, put her finger over her lips, and said, "Sssshhhhh."

Leaning in, she said, "Be quiet; maybe nobody noticed. This is not going to be good for your PR."

Looking over her head, I watched a male worker open the laundry room where the bathroom baskets were stored. Getting around Squeaks almost cost me a shower, but I caught him before he locked the door. Not stepping inside with him, I propped the door open, watching. I knew what happened when the door shut.

"What's your name?" he asked.

"James."

"I don't see a basket with your name on it. Let me see your wristband."

"I don't have one. See?" I said, holding out my arms.

"Why don't you have one? How are we supposed to know who you are?"

"I'm visiting, not here for long," I said, shrugging my shoulders.

"Uh-huh, whatever you say. You got thirty minutes. Turn the basket in at the desk when you're done."

With a towel over my shoulder and a little plastic basket no bigger than the crayon holder on the coffee table, I shut the door to my room with my free hand. Behind the saloon door to the bathroom, there wasn't enough room to move between the sink and shower, so I stripped down by the bed. First the shirt, then the shorts. By the time my briefs hit the floor, the door had burst open, and I fell backward on the bed, trying to cover up on the way down.

"Doors stay open. Is that clear?" boomed a male voice as the knob smacked the wall.

Before I could respond, he was gone. The walk to the shower using my clothes for cover offered more privacy than the shower itself. Everyone walking by could see right in without a curtain and with the mini swinging door facing the common area. Stooping in defeat, I let the warm water roll off my back. As steam swirled around me, sadness built within until the tears spilled over, dancing among the water droplets.

CHAPTER 12

Sliding the shower basket across the raised counter of the nurse's desk, the male worker snatched it from my hand without saying a word. Not wanting to engage the stare-down, I noticed the common area was abandoned except for a single soul. The woman with the bright cross shirt sat at a small table against the wall. She picked at her fingernails with an empty gaze and swayed back and forth. Anxious and alone, she needed a friend.

I plopped into the empty seat and broke her stare, and she slammed her hands to the table. When the shock wore off, her eyes winced at the rhythm of the second hand working its way around the clock on the wall. The spirit of fear had her tucked away. Somewhere behind her empty eyes hid the strong woman she was supposed to be.

Fear, however, was pacing between us like a starving lion claiming a fresh kill.

"Where's everyone at?" I asked with a smile, taunting the enemy.

"Smoke break," she said, examining her raw fingertips.

"You didn't want to go outside?"

"It took everything I had to come out of my room," she said, raising her hand to her mouth as her eyes became glossy, holding back tears.

"I love your shirt. So bright and colorful with the cross on the back. Is that from the church you go to?"

"Yes," she said, looking everywhere but at me. "I should be in church, but my husband dropped me off last night. He said we were going to dinner."

"Funny, my wife dropped me off here last night too. I wonder why—"

"No, no, no, no, it can't be," she said, exploding away from the table and onto her feet. "That girl, that girl right there. We rescued her last week. Why is she here?"

"What girl?" I asked, turning around to see everyone returning from the smoke break.

"The one in the ballcap, there in the front."

"Nia? She came in after me. She said she died in a ditch and asked if I had something to do with bringing her back to life. What do you mean you rescued her?"

With one arm wrapped around her midsection, she propped up her free hand to her mouth, shaking.

"My church rescues girls. Runaway girls and girls caught in human trafficking. We'll even buy them if needed and get them to safety by whatever means necessary. We have a ranch in West Texas where we take them to detox and recover, but she shouldn't be here. She ran away from our ranch after a couple of days, and we couldn't find her. How did she get here?"

Backing away, she turned and bolted across the room, disappearing into her room. The crowd filing in from the smoke break didn't bother sitting or hanging around. They moved through the room and formed a line like the one for breakfast. Joining them, Ma picked me out of the crowd and waved for me to come alongside her. We funneled down the empty hall, corralled like senseless animals. I wondered if the workers knew we were the sole survivors of the rapture. Maybe they knew beforehand and volunteered to keep us safe from the outside world until the second coming, and that's why the building was a maze. It must have been built to withstand the world's burning down.

Finding the same spot as earlier, Ma and the group took their seats, but I bypassed them and sat facing the floor-to-ceiling windows. The world outside still seemed alive and moving. The wind blew through the trees and kissed the tops of the shrubs. No one was outside the glass, though; everyone was gone. I wondered how much time had passed and how long until I could leave.

The weight of spending eternity locked within these walls began to smother what little joy I had left to give. Tears built over the untouched food tray as I pushed it aside and laid my head down. When the clutch of sadness released its grip enough for me to focus, my ears were filled with whispers storming the room.

I heard he's an oil tycoon.

No, he ran a company for an oil tycoon.

Yeah, he did run it, but there were explosions at the oil rigs that killed everyone.

I heard he tried to warn them, but he didn't make it in time. He watched it happen. Can you imagine?

That's why he's here. He watched them burn alive, and there was nothing he could do.

Sitting up with my head on a swivel, the whispers stopped. Everyone turned their eyes down, and no one said another word. Could it be true? I thought the explosion was at my house. What if they were right, and the same people who blew the oil rigs also came for my home? Now it made sense.

Throwing my food in the trash and shelving the tray, I took the first spot in line to leave. The young couple who had sat across the table from me at breakfast jumped in next. They both looked fresh out of high school. The dark-haired girl with olive skin even wore a T-shirt from my alma mater. Her boyfriend, with shoulder-length hair and plain tee, was doing pushups on the wall next to me.

"Don't worry. You're safe. I got your back," he said between reps.

Not sure what to say, the worker releasing us through the door broke the conversation, and I nodded in agreement as we stepped into the hallway. Returning to the common area, Ma grabbed my arm and said, "It's time to go. We have an appointment."

She walked us to a small classroom with a whiteboard on the front wall. Whitewashed wooden benches fastened to the walls ran along both sides of the room. Motioning for me to sit, she turned and left the room as the others arrived. On my right sat a mid-twenties metalhead wearing a black Hendrix shirt. With his glazed-over eyes and crazy hair pointing to the ceiling, I thought he was a famous musician. To my left, pinned against the back wall, sat a square-jawed man. Arms crossed and stiff as a board, except one tapping foot. He was filled with so much rage he could hardly keep it contained.

With everyone sitting along the walls, one last lady shut the door behind her. She limped to the front of the room in a dull blue dress that almost touched the floor. Reaching the front, she turned to address the room. With a quivering voice, she spoke and filled the whiteboard. She was undoubtedly from the world. She said the world says healing happens through your own hands and efforts. Self-healing, yoga, and meditation are the way to happiness. With simple breathing and self-exploration techniques, happy hormones were released for healing.

"You're missing the most important piece of the puzzle," I said, cutting her off.

"Raise your hand before you speak. You're disrupting the room," she said, waving her finger at me.

I raised my hand while spurting out, "What about God? Where do you think He fits on your whiteboard?"

"You can't raise your hand and speak at the same time. You wait until you're called on. Since you asked, though, God doesn't belong on my whiteboard. These are proven techniques that therapeutically work. God is a suggestion. A made-up idea no different than a unicorn."

"Then why are you so scared?"

"I'm sorry?" she asked, setting down her marker and removing her glasses.

"You've been trembling since you walked in here, like you're scared to death of us. If your techniques work so well, why are you so nervous? I don't even remember yesterday, and I'm not scared. God has a plan for everyone, and fear isn't part of any of them. He gives peace beyond understanding, so I guess you're right. He won't ever belong on your whiteboard."

"I think it's best if you leave my room sir," she said, pointing toward the door. "Now!"

"I'd love some fresh air. Thank you."

Stepping into the common area, the door spit me out next to the window where everyone went for their cigarettes. A list of names was taped to the wall next to the window, but mine was not one of them. Since the room was a mirror image of itself, I guessed another window was on the opposite side.

Following the curved counter around, Squeaks popped out of her room with a phone to her ear. "Yes, of course. Uh-huh, uh-huh. Hold on, he's right here." She leaned in with her hand over the phone and said, "It's my husband. Pretend to be my doctor, and tell him I can go home now."

If her husband had survived, maybe my wife had as well. I needed the phone. "If you do the same for me, you got a deal."

"Deal," she squeaked, jumping for joy and handing me the phone.

Clearing my throat, I took the phone. "Hello, sir. Your wife is fine to go home now. You can come and get her."

Tugging on my arm and giggling hysterically, she caused me to break character and burst out laughing with her.

"You're not her doctor. Put my wife back on the phone," said her irritated husband.

Handing the phone back with a shrug, she took it, chirped, "Bye," and hung up. "Here you go," she said. "Your turn."

I dialed my wife's number as the excitement built. Was she still alive? Had she made it to safety? Did she still remember me? Pushing send, my diaphragm clenched with anticipation as the phone rang.

"Hello," she answered in the same sweet, loving tone I remembered. Over her voice carried the sound of children playing in the background. She was alive, but where was she?

"Hi, honey," I said, smiling at Squeaks.

"How are you feeling?" she asked.

"Good, good. When are you coming to get me?"

"I haven't talked to the doctor yet, and you have to take your medicine."

"I'm fine, honey. When are you coming to get me?"

"I haven't talked to the doctor yet. I can't come get you."

"The doctor's right here, and she wants to talk to you. Hold on," I said, covering the phone and giggling as I passed it to Squeaks. "It's go time."

Grabbing the phone from my hand, "Hi!" she squealed with excitement. "No, I'm not a doctor. I'm a patient." After a brief pause, she shrugged and said, "Okay, it was so nice to meet you!"

Handing me the phone, Squeaks skipped away, full-on laughing. "That was not your doctor," said my wife firmly. "You need to take your medicine. They said you should be there for about seven days. I'll see you soon. I have to let you go now. Love you."

My, "I love you too, honey," was met with an echoing dial tone.

Setting the phone on the counter, I leaned, slipping into thought. I still didn't know where she was. She must have rescued the children in the background. She was keeping them safe. That's why she couldn't come to get me. The sound of the children's joy and laughter danced in my head. Of course, it had to be Disney World. The happiest place on earth. It all made perfect sense. She must have fled when the rapture happened and made it to safety there.

Knowing her, she was saving all the left-behind children she could grab on her way.

God knew the children not taken in the rapture would need a safe and joyous place to ride out the storm. He had been designing those theme parks all along to sustain us. I knew there was a reason they became a massive empire and took control of all their lifelines. Transportation, lodging, food, and even entertainment within the confines and control of their theme parks. We must be in Revelation now. The end times. Everyone got it wrong. The world may be falling apart and burning down, but God had another plan for His children. He would carry us through the flames so we never saw an ounce of pain or terror. Disney World: who would have thought? Why was I supposed to be here for seven more days, though?

"You need something?" boomed the voice of the cruel man behind the counter.

I shook my head no, unable to think of a response.

"Then get off the counter and find something to do."

Staring me down like he wanted a fight, I told myself it was a test and I shouldn't respond. They were pulling me into their games to ensnare me like the rest. I looked away and continued around the counter, returning to my original task. I had to find the window on the other side. Checking the list of names, mine was one of them. The window was closed, but I sat on the stool below and leaned on the small, protruding sill. Inside looked like some sort of control center. Computers and files lined the walls. A lady in scrubs sitting inside slid the window open.

"Yes, can I help you?" she asked, tapping her pen on the mug in front of her.

"I'm not sure. My name is on the wall out here. I'm not sure why."

"This is where you come for your medicine. Are you ready to start taking yours?"

"What is it? What's it for?"

"It's for sleep," she said, then rattled off some words that sounded like a foreign language.

"I was told I don't have to take any medicine if I don't want to."

"You're right. No one can force you, but don't you want to sleep?"

"Why do you want me to sleep? What's going to happen? What are y'all going to do to me?"

"Nothing. Nothing is going to happen to you, but you need your sleep."

"No thanks. You keep your pills," I said, standing to my feet.

Walking past an empty room that mimicked the one I had been kicked out of earlier, I followed the wall around the corner. The last one before the exit was a closed door with a narrow vertical window. The nameplate on the wall held a paper tag with a doctor's name. Every doorway had temporary paper labels. Even the emergency evacuation maps by the doors were paper. I was in a funhouse, and nothing was real. They could change whatever they wanted, whenever they wanted.

Glaring in the window, a hefty man wearing a black suit jacket and a crimson necktie stared back from behind a desk. Across from him sat a hunched-over lady, crying into her hands. Swinging the door open, I pinned my foot, so it wouldn't shut.

"Is this guy bothering you?" I asked the distressed lady.

She didn't look up or notice I was there, but the man rose to his feet. "You can't barge in here like that."

"I just did. I don't trust none of you. You all right,

ma'am?"

"She's fine. You need to leave."

"You a doctor?" I asked, poking at the sign outside the door.

"Yes, I'm the head doctor here."

"Good, we need to talk," I said, pointing back and forth between us.

"You can wait your turn like everyone else," he said, coming around the desk, tie flapping, to shoo me out the door.

"Fair enough," I said, backing away. "But you have a lot of explaining to do."

As the door shut behind me, I remembered passing by the refrigerator, and my stomach was growling. I wondered what was in it, but taped to the door was another paper sign that said, *Do not open.* Loving your neighbor and respecting authority was one thing, but being held prisoner was another. In defiance, I thought I'd help myself. Consider it the spoils of war. Surprisingly, it was empty except for a handful of white paper-wrapped balls on the top shelf.

"They're oranges," whispered Squeaks, inches from

my ear.

Almost smacking my head on the door in shock, she let out her high-pitched giggle. "You shouldn't be in there. You're supposed to ask the workers."

"Why would I wait on them? These have to be for us, or they wouldn't be out here." Grabbing one for myself, "You want one?"

"Oh goody, goody, goody. Yes," she said, clapping her hands and bouncing like there were springs under her feet.

"Why are they wrapped up in little baggies?" I asked, tearing into mine.

"They don't want people like us touching them. You know, some of these other people don't bathe for weeks. They don't want those nut jobs licking each one and putting them back. You never know with some of these weirdos," she said, holding her unpeeled orange. She sank her teeth in and took off a chunk, peel, and all. Grinning from ear to ear, juice spilled from both sides of her mouth and dripped from her chin.

"Look, it's time to go outside," I said, walking around her toward the large crowd huddled by the door. Tossing the peel in the trash can by the fountain drink machine, I joined the group next to Ma. Before one of the staff made it to the front to let us out, one of the women rushed around the corner in a panic.

"They won't let her go out. They're trying to keep her in her."

"Who?" asked Ma.

"The young woman who came in last night. The one with the hat. See, they have her cornered in the chair over there. I tried to grab her, but she didn't understand me, and they ran me off."

"Why is she freaking out?" I asked, turning to Ma.

"That's what they do in these kinds of places. They prey on the young ones. Separate them from the group and do what they want. Who's going to believe her? Who's going to believe us for that matter? Everyone thinks we're crazy, remember? We're trapped."

Pushing through the crowd, I saw her sitting in the common area. Head down, she was cowering under the male staff member who barked at me every chance he got. *He feeds on fear. The same fear trying to take hold of me.* With my heart pounding, I got within a few feet of her before the man put his arm up to stop me.

"Hey, come on outside with us."

She heard my voice and peeked from under the corner of her hat bill. Her eyes were red, and tears rolled down her cheeks. She was scared and confused.

"Come on. Let's go outside."

"She's staying with us. Get back in line."

"Why?"

"Mind your business and go get in line. Don't make me tell you again," he growled.

I extended my hand to her while staring fear in the eyes, asking her to come outside with the group again. Feeling surrounded, I turned to see a handful of the women encircling us.

Ma stepped forward, took her hand, and said, "Come on, dear. Let's go."

The group surrounded her, and the huddle moved toward the door. Leaving me to guard the rear, I followed a few steps behind.

The doors opened, pulling us out like a vacuum. The women walked to the far end of the courtyard, still in protection mode. When they reached the wrought-iron bars, Ma peeled off and returned in my direction.

"Come here," she said, with a smile on her face. "That was brave of you back there. I didn't think you could stand your ground. That was amazing."

"Nah," I said, sitting on the edge of the small wall lining the sidewalk. "I was glad y'all showed up when you did. I wasn't sure what was about to happen."

She took her shoes off and ran her toes through the grass, looking over the field beyond the fence. "I need to get out of here and go see my horses. I love riding horses. Take off your shoes," she said, pointing to my feet. "It's relaxing."

I did as she said and planted my feet among the soft blades. We both stared off into the horizon, not saying a word. The wind melodically quieted my fears. One by one, people joined us, barefoot on the wall, until the worker by the door yelled it was time to go in. My spirit was renewed enough to go another round. Ma still hadn't said a word, but I knew she was on the right side of the rapture. That was good enough for me. It only takes a mustard seed of faith to change the world.

As the group moved through the doors, I abandoned them for my room. Next to my door, though, was another room with its own paper name tags. I had to say hello. Frigid air met me at the threshold, seeping from the darkness. Some might say it was a warning sign, but I had souls to save, so I continued easing into the room. Three steps in and ten degrees colder, my breath rose to the ceiling. Eyes adjusting enough to see the faint outline of the first empty bed, my heartbeat quickened. The room was a mirror image of mine, the exact opposite in the physical realm and spiritual. Something evil was lurking in the shadows.

I reached the wooden shelves for support and was knocked off balance. A sharp blow ripped through my chest like a dull arrow, and I couldn't move further. Vision now cutting through the darkness, a man's silhouette on the second bed became focused. Crouched in the corner like a predator, he studied me the whole time.

"I wanted to say hi since you didn't come outside with us," I said.

He unfolded his posture and lay on his back with hands behind his head with elbows pointing out, like someone without a care in the world. He threw one foot over his knee, tapping the air as he said, "There's a reason for that. I wanted to be alone; you shouldn't be here."

"It's not good to be alone. God designed us to interact with not only Him but other people." With no response, a few silent seconds passed like hours. "Why are you in here?" I asked.

"I did a very, very bad thing," he said as his bouncing foot stopped. "I can't control my rage. My demons take over, and I become a passenger."

"That may be so, but your demons are no match for my God. He forgives and heals those who ask and accept Him. You can be set free."

Rising to a sitting position, his hands clenched the bedside, and his bare feet gripped the floor. He was hanging on, fighting the urge to lunge at me as his knee violently bounced. His head rose, revealing the whites of his bloodshot eyes. An arrogant grin formed across his face, and his eyes were consumed by darkness.

"You should leave us be," he growled, fighting through multiple voices. "Or we might use you for our next toy."

"Yes, our next toy," hissed another voice. "There's no fight left in this one."

"You have no authority here. Not over him or me, in Jesus's name. I'll leave you alone, but that doesn't mean I won't be praying for you."

Warmth returned to my body upon exiting the darkness, and I looped into my room. The place was a playground for evil spirits. So many weak and lost people for them to feed on. My room may have been the only safe space in the building. I thought about staying in there for good. Who would help all the poor souls, though? If not me, then who? It was my role in the new world after the rapture. I wasn't so sure I had signed up for the task at hand. I'd never thought of myself as a warrior before.

CHAPTER 13

The dinner line formed, but I hung back. Jesus took naps, and now I knew why. Walking between the spiritual realm and this world was no easy task. Even when the people were silent, the groaning of their spirits fighting against their ancient enemies was overwhelming. With everyone outside the door, I prayed my way around the common area. Prayers for protection. Prayers for healing. Prayers for forgiveness and freedom.

When the crowd returned from their meal, I sat at one of the small tables for two. With my back to the wall, I was anxiously waiting for someone, any one of them, to walk through the door and get smacked in the face by the Holy Spirit. With the excitement of a prank-playing child, the unbridled anticipation had me laughing and holding my breath. They slowly moved through the door to their rooms or the sitting area. When the last person entered, I knew my prayers didn't work. At least not yet.

Like an ant farm, they marched in lines wherever told. The smoke break was no different. They ran to the window to grab their cigarettes, then raced to the doors behind me to go out. This wasn't by human control, though. The spirit of addiction had a hold on them. Not even a vicious or forceful grip. No, this embrace was sweet deception, a false comforter. No need to seek the Lord when the numbness of pills and nicotine produced a temporary sense of peace. The pills always run out, though, and the cigarette packs fall empty.

Even the former pastor I spoke with this morning walked by, Bible in one hand, cigarettes in the other. Saying, "Praise Jesus, it's time for a smoke," while waving the Bible high above his head. At least it was a step in the right direction, and he might find his fire again.

With my head bowed, the clamoring faded from the doorway behind me. The sweet voice of an elderly lady broke the silence.

"Hi there. Would you like to play some cards with me?"

A rather tall woman with long gray hair towered over the table. Cards in hand, she pulled the chair out and sat before I could answer. Pink framed glasses dangled from her neck, hung by a sparkling chain of plastic beads.

"Well?" she said, sliding the cards out of the box.

"Yeah, I'd love to. But numbers are hard for me right now."

"I can hardly see them myself," she said. "How about we play memory match with the shapes?"

"Sure, but I can't even remember yesterday so you're probably going to win."

"Oh, this will be perfect then." Her eyes lit up. "This is what my doctor makes me play for my own memory. Maybe it will help yours too."

"Maybe so," I said, reaching for the cards. "I'll shuffle."

With the table now covered in face-down cards, we played through a couple of rounds in silence. Her posture and poetic hand movement told a tale of wealth and stature. If twenty years were removed along with the cards, we'd be sitting in front of fine china, sipping tea, and discussing her vacation homes. The way her weathered hands searched the table for pairs revealed a long and comfortable life.

She put her glasses on without either of us matching a pair yet. To help, I suppose. She sat there, concentrating on what card to pick up for a minute. Then she turned her eyes to me and reached out her hand. "I'm Mary Lou," she said. "What's your name?"

"James. Nice to meet you," I replied, shaking her hand.

"It's always nice to know your opponent's name before destroying their pride," she said with a grin. "James, you seem like a nice young man, but I don't take prisoners."

With that, she matched almost half the table's worth of cards. Stacking them in neat little piles in front of her. "Why are you here, James?" she asked intently, pausing the game.

"I'm not sure. How about you? You seem like a sweet lady."

"My kids say I'm old and crazy. I'm fine on my own, you know. Between you and me, they want to put me in a home and take my money. I keep telling them I'm not dead yet. Greedy little bastards can't wait a few more years, I guess. They told these people my memory was going, and I was not taking my medications. Both are true, but they shouldn't have locked me in here." She looked around to ensure no one was listening, cards shifting from hand to hand. "You know what happens when I don't take my medicine?" she asked, pulling her glasses down to the edge of her nose.

"What's that?"

"I see things. Things most people will never see. Shouldn't see for that matter."

The doors crashed open behind me. The smoking crowd entered the common area, and Mary Lou regained her proper sitting posture. A loud, unnerving thud vibrated from the floor behind me. A short scream followed by agonizing cries and whimpers burst through the room. A young woman tossed and turned on the floor in what looked to be unbearable pain.

"She does that every day for attention," Mary Lou scoffed. "Kids nowadays will do anything for attention."

"She probably doesn't have any friends. Don't you know what it's like to be all alone and afraid?"

I walked over and stood above the writhing girl. Rolling between two workers and me, her cries intensified. They bent to her and attempted lifting her from the ground to no avail as she wiggled loose. The irritated workers were now more intimidating than helpful, so I kneeled in front of her on the floor, motioning for them to stop. Hands over both her ears, she still tossed back and forth, with her eyes sealed shut while crying out. I gently placed my hand on her arm, and she flinched and pulled back. When my hand stayed on her arm, she peeked from one eye, and the rolling fit ended.

"Hi there. I'm playing cards with my friend Mary Lou. I'll bring a chair over for you to join us when you're done here. Whenever you're ready, we'll be waiting for you."

When I got to my feet, the staff had already gone about their business. The crowd of half-sedated gawkers dispersed while I grabbed a chair from the adjacent table and sat across from Mary Lou again.

"Why on earth would you ask her to play cards with us?" asked Mary Lou, leaning over the table. "If she were any younger, I'd throw her over my knee and teach her a lesson."

Realizing no one was around, the young lady sat up and wiped the tears from her cheeks. She pretended to dust off her homemade capris and joined us at the table.

Mary Lou turned cold and silent, nose to the wall, pretending not to see our guest.

"Glad you could join us. I'm James, and this is Mary Lou. What's your name?"

"Jesse," she said, staring at the floor.

"I think we should start over. Don't you, Mary Lou? Mary Lou? Let's start over so our new friend can join us."

"I know how to shuffle," said Jesse, now making eye contact.

"Here," said Mary Lou, shoving the scattered cards toward Jesse. "We're playing a memory match. The shapes only, not the numbers."

"Doesn't that make the game a little too easy?"

I watched Mary Lou's nostrils flare as if her intellect had taken a fatal blow from a peasant and braced for the worst. Raising her chin to the insult, she stared down her pointy nose and through her reading glasses for a second in thought.

"Yes, it does make it easy," said Mary Lou. "But James here isn't good with numbers. I, on the other hand, am great with numbers."

"You two should play," I said, jumping up. "I need a

break anyway. Y'all have fun."

A small group lounged around the sitting area, watching a television hanging high on the wall. I grabbed an empty chair from one of the tables and found an open space by Ma. Some people were coloring crazy hard pictures that looked like animals but had a million little spaces to fill in. A thousand-piece puzzle took up the other half of the coffee table. It was the kind with pieces so small they made ordinary people question their sanity.

Ma, however, was staring at the television, not paying attention. She didn't mind when I broke her concentration with questions. Like why were there so many intricate coloring books instead of easy ones and why tiny puzzles with millions of pieces? She chuckled and shrugged her shoulders.

"It's almost like they want to keep us frustrated and crazy, isn't it?" she said. "If you haven't noticed, nothing about this place is made to help people get better. The longer you're here, the more pills you pop and the more money they make. This place is an evil machine. I've never been religious, but it's hard to sleep in a place like this." Ma leaned in close. "See that white-haired lady sitting by herself against the wall over there? She claims to be a high priestess of a wiccan coven. I tend to believe her with how the air grows cold when she's close. That, and because she has fangs, of course."

I hadn't seen her until now, but sure enough, there she was. Observing the room from a small table off to the side. White stringy hair hugged her pale face and crawled over her broad shoulders like a briar thicket. Her head spun in our direction like she heard Ma talking. I was all too familiar with the black, hollow eyes now fixated on us. The evil attached to her was dark and tangible, circulating in and around her body. Ma couldn't see beyond the natural, though. She also couldn't see the child of God behind her eyes, trying to find a way back to the light.

"How come I haven't seen her yet?" I asked.

"She got here a few days ago. Right after me, in fact. I don't think she's gone to eat once yet, and, except for the smoke breaks, she has stayed in her room the rest of the time."

"I'm going to say hi."

"You're braver than any of us. Good luck," said Ma as I walked away.

Her bottomless eyes fixated on my every step as I got close. Screams of sorrow and weeping emanated from the depths of her soul, and I could hear God's child fighting and searching to escape her tormenter. I sat across from her, and the hairs raced up my arms and neck as her posture stiffened. The one in control didn't like my intrusion.

"You looked lonely, so I thought I'd come say hi."

A shallow growl rumbled from her chest like a dog guarding a bone. The wrinkles on her forehead clenched, and her hands clamped to the table's edge.

"It's okay. Make all the noise you want. I didn't come to talk to you anyway. I want to talk to that sweet lady you're hiding from me. The one Jesus died for. She's in there. I can see her."

Her head cocked to the side, then silence. The depth of darkness in her eyes reflected the sad toll of a lost and twisted life. She stood, still gripping the table. With a snap of her wrists, the table jumped, and she disappeared through the doorway to her room.

After a few minutes, my pounding heart subsided, and I joined the others in the sitting area.

"Interesting. What did you say to her?" Ma asked.

Still processing, I didn't respond to Ma's prying. My eyes were glued to the television on the wall. A handful of conversations were happening around us, and no one paid attention to them but me. Voices were coming from the television, hundreds of them. Layering over each other, feeding off one another. Amid the cruel and remorseless heckling were cries of terror, calling out from the abyss. The abusers were taunting and laughing at the torture their victims were enduring. The torment was unbearable. I ran to my room for peace, wondering how no one else heard what I was hearing.

After staring at the ceiling for a while, the noise drifting from the common area died down, and darkness peered through the cracks of the thin plastic blinds. Emerging from my shelter once again, the whole place was dim and almost vacant. The high-school-aged couple from the cafeteria played cards at one of the small tables against the wall. Without invitation, I pulled a chair up to their table.

"You want to play next round?" asked the young man.

"No thanks. I'm not good with numbers anymore."

"What brought you here?" asked his girlfriend.

"I'm not sure yet. All I remember is my wife dropping

me off. What about y'all?"

"We checked ourselves in for the weekend," he said, flipping over the last card on the river.

"We do it for some extra cash from time to time," she said, studying the cards in her hand.

"What do you mean 'extra cash'?" I asked, turning my chair for a better view of the room.

Laying his hand down, "Two pairs, pay up," he said with a grin. "We're here to watch over the patients. A nonprofit organization pays us to check in for the weekend at different facilities to keep an eye on things. You would be surprised what goes on in places like this."

"Thousands of girls go missing from facilities like this one every year. They dope them up on meds. The lights go out, then, poof, they disappear like magic. When the family comes looking, they're told their daughter or sister checked themself out. Never to be seen again. Girls without families are the easiest targets. If they're eighteen, people can check themselves out so the cops can't do anything." Her eyes glossed over with anger as she collected the cards on the table.

"Human trafficking thrives because of places like this.

Even if someone in here witnessed something, think about it: Who would believe a crazy person? No offense, but between the meds and the crazy, no one would believe them even if they could remember what happened. We try to stay up all night to make sure nothing fishy happens. Sometimes we make it, sometimes we don't, but we still get paid," said the boyfriend.

"I'll be up all night, don't worry. What about that guy sitting by himself?" I asked, pointing toward the far side of the room.

"He tries to stay up all night too. We're not sure why though."

"I'm going to go keep him company. No sense in him sitting alone," I said, leaving the table.

Walking up from behind, he looked like a linebacker. His shoulders were as broad as the chair, and his head looked like a football helmet.

"Hi. I'm James," I said, sitting beside him.

"Richard," he said with a nod. "Nice to meet you."

His eyes didn't fully open, but he cracked a slight grin because of the company, I think. In full view of the rest of him, it was a wonder the chair supported his frame. In another lifetime, he would no doubt have struck fear in any opponent on the field.

"What brings you here, Richard?"

"Well, I'm trying to get free," he said.

"Free from what?"

"Addiction, depression, anger. You name it, I'm fighting it."

"That's a lot of fighting, but I guess we all have our battles. You want to talk about it?"

"Where should I start?" he said, shrugging his sedan-sized shoulders. "I had a college scholarship for football. On the last game of my senior year in high school, I tore my ACL. It was so bad I had to have multi-ligament reconstruction, and my scholarship was dropped before I got off the operating table."

"Sorry to hear that. Must have been disappointing."

"I'm just getting warmed up," he said, propping his leg on the coffee table. He rolled the leg of his shorts up, revealing the remains of what used to be a kneecap. "Ten years of agonizing pain and seven surgeries later, I still can't walk right."

"I guess that's where the anger comes from then, huh?"

"And the addiction," he said, crossing his arms. "I made the mistake of returning to the same surgeon because he said he could fix it and make it right. Each time it got worse instead of better. The more pain, the more pills I popped. I didn't set out to get addicted to painkillers, but here I am."

"Do you believe in God, Richard?"

"Ha, God. Not sure I do anymore. I did find one of the best orthopedic surgeons in the country, though. Sent him my records. He said it was the worst he'd seen in twenty-five years of work. That's really why I'm here. He said he'd take my case, so I checked myself here. I want my life back. I want to beat the addiction and depression I'd been battling before the surgery. A clean slate. Know what I mean?"

"I do, and this might sound crazy, but I'd like to pray with you. If you don't mind. What could it hurt, right?"

"Nothing, I suppose. I'm not praying with you, though," he said, waving his pointer finger. "I haven't prayed in years.

Rubbing the palms of my hands together, I kneeled beside his chair. With my head bowed, I cupped his knee and began to pray. I prayed aloud for the healing and restoration of his knee and spirit in Jesus's name for peace beyond measure to replace anger and a tidal wave of joy to subdue depression. I prayed he would forgive the doctor who left him like this. As I continued praying, heat radiated around and through my hands. Like the Holy Spirit was caressing my hands, healing not only his knee but also his heart.

When my prayer ceased and I returned to my chair, I could see faint streaks where tears ran down his cheeks. "Thank you," he said. "I think I'm going to do some praying of my own."

Excusing himself, he limped to his nearby room.

My younger card-playing friends must have called it a night. It looked like I was alone again. Grabbing one of the last wrapped oranges from the refrigerator, I enjoyed it in my room. After all, fruit is the Lord's candy.

I tossed myself onto the bed. It felt good to spread God's love, but my celebration was cut short by a wall-shaking snore from the bed beside me. Jumping into the air, I launched the orange out of shock, smacking the blinds and making an awful noise on its way to the floor. The snoring continued. Maybe I was in the wrong room. Fleeing through the door, I checked the paper name tags by the door. Sure enough, there was my name, and underneath it was another.

I slid my paper label from the holder and returned to the room, entering the bathroom. Blood spots smeared on the counter left a trail to a syringe in the trash can. I wondered how he had snuck it in. They were thorough when they checked me in. Piece by piece, I ripped my name tag to little shreds and flushed it down the toilet. No wristband, no name on the door. I no longer existed. Maybe I could escape.

An argument erupted in the common area, and from the bathroom, it was louder than my new roommate's snoring. Through the darkness, two men were struggling over a mattress outside one of the rooms. Now ten feet away, I could tell one was a staff member, a grown man, and the other was a tall, lanky teenager.

"Hey, what's going on here?" I asked, getting closer.

"Doesn't concern you," said the man in scrubs, trying to rip the mattress away.

"I think it does. He's a kid, and you're a grown man."

"He can't bring his mattress outside the room."

"Why not? It's not hurting anyone."

"It's against the rules, that's why not. Now mind your business."

"Where I'm from we have a different set of rules. The kind that says a grown man doesn't mess with a kid. I suggest you let go and walk away."

"Or what?" he asked, releasing the mattress and throwing his hands out to his sides.

"You really want to find out?"

Dropping his hands, he shook his head and walked off. I turned and saw why he had given up. Heads were popping in and out of doorways like curious gophers. The wiry teen wrestled the mattress to the floor and disappeared into his room, returning with a pillow. He crawled under the burlap sack of a blanket and hid half his face, leaving nothing but his eyes and matted hair exposed. I laid on the cold, hard floor and used my hands for a pillow, staring at the ceiling.

"So, what brings you to the hallway?" I asked, propping one foot on top of the other. A few minutes went by with no response. I glanced at him, and his face disappeared under the cover. So much fear for such a young kid who hadn't even been out in the real world yet.

"I'm staying right here with you. You'll be safe. Don't worry."

"Are you scared, too?" he asked after a few minutes of silence.

"Not at all. Why?" I said, still staring at the ceiling.

"Because you're shaking."

"That's because I don't have a blanket. It's freezing down here."

"Okay. Yeah, I guess that makes sense. Thanks for helping me out."

"Why were you fighting so hard to sleep on the ground and not in your room?"

"I felt trapped, and I panicked. They put some other dude in there with me. How am I supposed to sleep in a tiny room next to some crazy old man who talks to himself all night?"

"You're right about that for sure. You want me to find somewhere else to hang out?"

"No. Please, uh, if you could stay until I fall asleep, that'd be cool."

"Sounds good. I'll hang out for a bit."

Laying on the cold ground for what seemed like forever, my new friend was sound asleep. I sat up, facing the glass door calling my name. Worth a shot, but it was still locked. Walking past the mattress on the floor, the girl from the card game waved me to the table where she sat.

"Jesse, wasn't it?" I asked, taking a seat.

"Yes. Why are you still awake?"

Her voice was dainty, cartoonish even. I hadn't noticed earlier, but it sounded odd coming from someone of her age and solid frame. It reminded me of a cartoon mouse.

"There's too much going on to sleep. How about you?"

"I can't sleep either. Sometimes an hour or two is all I get. That was awful nice of you to help that kid out over there. You must have a few of your own."

"I, I don't remember. I know my wife dropped me off here. I can't remember anything before, though."

"So, you don't remember why you're here?" she asked.

"No, I sure don't. Do you know why you're in here?"

"Yeah, I do. I'm not proud of it," she said, looking down at her twiddling fingers. "I was kicked out of my house by my stepdad. My mom didn't say a word. She watched me back out of the driveway. I've been homeless for weeks and wanted someplace to sleep beside my car. I ran out of money for food, so I checked myself here. They'll probably kick me out of here soon. My mom's insurance will run out at some point."

"Things will get better," I said, patting the tops of her balled-up hands.

"I don't think they will," she said, bursting into tears.

"Let's pray. Will you pray with me?"

She shifted her hands across the table, and I grasped her hands in prayer. We bowed our heads as I prayed over her life. She sobbed violently as I prayed for healing in her family, body, and mind. She was alive for a reason, and God hadn't even begun working miracles through her yet. Whatever brought her here made her strong enough to save someone else. Opening my eyes, I released her hands. Drawing back, she buried her head in her arms.

The air turned bitter, as if life itself were sucked from the room. A dark, faceless figure leaned over the counter at the worker's station. Shrouded in black, the only spot of color was the white square at the collar. The kind pastors wear. Whatever that thing was, a pastor it was not.

Leaning arrogantly in our direction, I heard it say, "I never thought I'd see the day."

What day? I asked myself.

"The day someone would think they could save a soul I've already taken. I worked hard for that one. You can't have her."

Her crying stopped, and the room was silent. She was face down and motionless. The stranger at the counter was gone. Slowly, she lifted her head. Her empty and emotionless eyes stared through me. A faint spiderweb of fine cracks snaked across her face from ear to ear, then crawled throughout her forehead. Popping and crackling, the faint lines became deeper and more pronounced, like the face of an antique porcelain doll. She opened her mouth to scream, but her face shattered and cascaded to the floor, followed by the rest of her fractured body.

Taking a knee, I ran my hand through the mound of broken pieces. As I lifted a handful, the fragile pieces turned to ash and sifted through my fingertips, dissolving into the air. Within a single moment, she was gone. Alone on the floor, I wept and prayed, searching for answers.

CHAPTER 14

I sat and watched the cleaning staff wipe the counters, empty trash cans, and put the room together again as best they could. While they were finishing up, a man with a dangling badge forced a steel cart through the doors. He heaved a full coffee dispenser onto the counter and disappeared the way he came. First, in line, I filled one of the white foam cups to the brim and returned to my seat. I enjoyed the last few minutes of peace sipping coffee before the hoards piled out of their rooms.

"Mr. James. Mr. James, it's time for your blood work. You need to come with us," said a man in scrubs from across the room.

A small group of patients was gathered by the doors. He knew my name, so I thought it was safe. Unless God wanted them to know it, no one would have known my name without my ID bracelet or name on the door. I thought it was my ticket to freedom. The last to join the group, we were led through the doors, down the hall, and stopped in a single-file line before we got to another room. One by one, people disappeared into the doorway and returned a few moments later to wait some more. With one person in front of me, I could see a doctor's table and two people in long white coats extracting blood from the arm of a timid woman.

Putting a cotton ball and a small band-aid on her arm, the man helped her off the table. Holding a clipboard, his female coworker called, "Next." The man in front of me slid onto the table. "What's your name?" she asked.

"James," he said.

I knew it. This was my chance to escape. When our escort turned his head, I snuck along the wall and disappeared around the corner. Out of sight, I took off, jogging toward the end of the hall. Locked. A few feet from the dead end was an open door to a dark room. Flipping the light switch revealed a few chairs and barren walls. It was one of the intake rooms.

A few minutes into kicking back with my feet propped up, a frantic worker smacked the door frame. "There you are. Had us scared to death. Come on, it's time for your blood work. You can't be running off like that."

Not the escape I had expected, but after blood work, I received a personal escort back to the living area. Pouring another cup of coffee, I returned to my open seat against the wall. The room was filled with movement and conversation as the rising sun pierced the skylights. The promise of a new day.

The white-haired witch, or high priestess as she called herself, lumbered from her room toward the coffee. Her head snapped back and forth in short bursts as people moved around her. It might be from the meds, but she looked scared and alone. When she tried to slink back into the darkness of her room, I tapped the table and invited her to sit.

"Come on, join me. Have a seat."

She paused in the doorway, looked into the darkness, and then back at me as she pulled the chair away from the table and sat.

"Good morning," I said, raising my cup. Her head

jerked erratically from me to the room, then back to me. Each time her attention landed on me, a slight smile broke through her cold face as I made small talk. She was unaware of the crowd forming behind her for the first smoke break of the day, and God handed me the perfect joke to break through her defenses.

"Do you like jokes?" I asked, setting my empty cup on the table. Her eyes showed interest, and her attention lingered on me instead of shifting again. "I'll take that as a yes. There's a Bible story about a group of religious leaders dragging a woman by her hair to the feet of Jesus. Do you know that one?" A healthy look of shock and curiosity stared back at me, but no answer. "So anyway, they threw her at Jesus's feet and said she was caught in adultery, demanding him to do something about it. Instead of condemning her, he said whoever hadn't sinned should cast the first stone. None of them could because everyone sins at some point. God still loves all of us, though. Anyway, here's the good part. Jesus kneeled, and while he wrote in the dirt, the crowd began to leave one by one. Now, a good friend of mine thinks he wrote *forgiven*, or *forgiveness*, for the lady. I've also been told he may have been drawing tally marks. Counting the sins of those who wanted to stone her. You know what I think he wrote?"

Eyes wide, she shook her head no.

Pretending to write on the tabletop, I said, "I think he bent over and wrote, *It's time for a smoke break.*" Then I pointed behind her. She turned to see the crowd walking through the doors, cigarettes in hand, and let out a quick, stifled laugh. Her fangs flashed before her hand could hide her smile. I had thought Ma was joking about the fangs. Shaking her head with a hint of joy, she grabbed her pack of smokes from the window and joined the crowd outside.

As the last few people made it through the doors, the noise dissipated with them. With no more coffee or people to keep me occupied, I rested my head on the table. About to doze off, a familiar mousy voice cut through the silence. It was Jesse, standing a few feet from the table.

"How is this possible? Last night, you disappeared," I said, jumping to my feet.

Her eyes welled up, and she tried to find the words to speak. "I couldn't do it," she said through the tears.

"Couldn't do what? I don't get it."

"I was going to kill myself last night, but I couldn't

do it," she said, using her sleeve to catch the tears. "I had it all planned out."

"What are you talking about?"

"I was waiting for everyone to sleep, then I was going to hang myself. But you were still awake and sat with me," she said, bursting into tears.

"I still don't get it. I watched you shatter to pieces and disappear last night. I thought you were gone," I said, reaching out to comfort her.

"I almost was," she murmured into my shoulder. "When you fell asleep while praying for me, I went to my room to end it. I was twisting the sheet into a noose, and your words kept playing in my head. I fell to my knees and prayed for the rest of the night. I've never prayed before."

Her warm tears soaked through my shirt as I told God how confusing this was, but also how grateful I was that He had saved her. Break time was over, and Ma was the first to join us as the other patients returned. Soon a whole group was comforting her, and I faded into the background. From a distance, I could see the love and compassion surrounding her. Even the supposed witch was consoling her. Proof that God uses anyone He chooses for

His work. I guessed it was His way of showing the enemy who was boss.

The line formed for breakfast, and I hung at the back. I was trying to grasp everything, so a bit of space was a welcome relief. After weaving through the food line, my hope of finding an abandoned corner fell short. Ma and Squeaks were on their feet, waving me in like a first-place runner. Sitting next to Ma, she and Squeaks dove in for more details. Excitement whirled about Jesse making it through the night. They poked and prodded. Without answering, I nodded along, pretending to listen.

Nia was sitting in her spot across from us. Picking at her food, she wasn't interested in the conversation. I shifted around in my seat, avoiding eye contact and discussion, and saw the man assigned to the bed beside mine walk by. He sat a row behind us and as far from everyone as possible. Intrigued, I watched as he crouched over his tray, held his fork like a shovel, and devoured everything within seconds. His posture and speed suggested he had spent a reasonable amount of time behind bars. Ma and the gang seemed to be getting along great. They made up a good-sized group, chatting, laughing, and supporting each other. My new roommate and the young lady across from me were singled out and alone. Always go for the one. *Leave the ninety-nine and go find the one,* reverberated through the room, highlighting the two lost souls that needed help. As much as I needed a break—some peace and quiet—my mission came first.

Moving to the row behind us, I sat across from my new roommate. Confused, he clenched his fork like I was about to steal his empty tray. "Come sit over there with us," I said, pointing toward the group.

"I'm good, man," he said, dropping the fork to his empty tray.

"We'd really like you to join us though. You're done eating. What do you have to lose?"

After a few minutes and rounds of persuasion, he agreed to sit with us. Nia's eyes widened from across the table when he sat beside me.

"Come on, you two. Since we're together, I'm going to say a prayer for us," I said, reaching for both their hands on the table. Neither said a word, but his eyes ballooned wider than hers. "I'll make it quick, promise," I said, tapping the table.

They extended their hands, and I took hold as we bowed our heads. Launching into prayer, I covered everything from healing their past to breaking bondages, and blessings for their future. After a few minutes of intense prayer, I said, "Amen." Both still looked shocked, but Nia was the first to break the silence with a glistening in her eyes. She said no one had ever prayed for her before. In the village where she had grown up as a child, God wasn't spoken of often. On occasion, people came through who looked like me talking about all the beautiful things this God could do, but then they left. Everything always went back to the way it was. I sat in awe, asking questions and listening as she walked through how she came to the U.S. The glistening in her eyes at the start of her testimony may have been pain, but by the end, they were tears of joy, because she was here and alive.

When she finally finished talking, I noticed the entire table was silent and in awe of her story. Nia dried her eyes, and everyone got up, tossing their trays to leave. Nia walked off, and Ma grabbed my arm, spinning me around.

"What was that?" she asked, not letting go of my arm.

"What was what?" I replied, trying to yank my arm free.

"You two were sitting there carrying on a conversation like it was no big deal."

"I know. Her story was amazing. Wasn't it?"

"Her story?" Ma said. "What story? None of us understood a single word of what you two were saying. None of it. What language was that?"

"You're losing it, Ma. We were speaking English, same as you and I are right now."

"No, you weren't. It didn't sound like anything we'd ever heard before. On top of that, she hasn't spoken to anyone since she got here. Even the staff can't get her to talk."

Finally freeing my arm, I shrugged it off and headed for the door where the last of the line was leaving. Funneling through the cold, sterile hallway, we were dumped back into the common area. One of the staff members caught me before disappearing into my room. She invited me to join her class, which started in a few minutes, and even walked me to her room. I couldn't pass up the opportunity. She knew my name, so she must have chosen me for a reason.

We were the last to walk into the room, and there was one empty schoolroom desk that she ushered me to after closing the door behind us. Taking her place at the front, she looked like a teacher. The badge dangling from her Disney princess lanyard hung below her salt and pepper hair. In place of scrubs were slacks and a button-down blouse. Not at all what the other staff wore, looked, or acted like. On the side wall of the room was a second door. Of course, the lanyard should have given it away. This was my ticket out. She was the key for me to see my wife again. That's why she had pulled me in the room. I had to get past this level and through the second door. It must lead to the secret passage where the Secret Service escort was waiting to sneak me out.

The teacher opened her bag and pulled out prints of artwork by famous artists. Some were black and white line drawings, others were colorful abstract images. She taped them to the whiteboard, explained how she was trying something new, and wanted us to pick our favorite. After choosing, she wanted us to tell everyone why we chose it. The selection process started on the opposite side of the room. I was surrounded by familiar faces but couldn't remember how long we'd been trapped. How many years had passed since we had seen our families? Moving through Squeaks, the preacher, and a few more, the choice finally landed on me. With so much at stake, I had to guess right. The one with the melting clock could be the correct answer because it was time to leave. Too obvious, though. Scanning from picture to picture, they each shouted a thousand hidden meanings, fighting to convince me which was correct. In a panic, I picked the most simplistic. The one not screaming.

"The picture with all the tiny feathers making up one big wing or whatever it is."

"And why do you like it the best?" she asked.

"The worldly way to say it is birds of a feather flock together. I see a group of unique people, like us here in the room, united and part of one big family."

"How so?"

"We're all God's children. That makes us family, and we're all stronger together."

"Interesting thought process. I like it."

The side door didn't fly open, and confetti didn't fall from the ceiling like I had hoped. Round one was over, and I was stuck. There was a good chance my wife didn't remember me anymore, and the longer I was stuck, the chance became more of a fact. The teacher moved to round two after telling us which picture she liked and why. For this round, she turned on the television and clicked through options until she landed on YouTube. I remembered YouTube. I knew they'd stand the test of time.

"This round," she explained, "each of you will pick a song, and we'll listen to thirty seconds of it."

While this seemed interesting, it was apparent we weren't being tested. At least not this round. Hanging my head, I stared at the mystery door as the song choices ran through the room. Ma picked a nineties country song, and the old preacher picked a piece of even older Christian music. So old, the video crackled in black and white as the choir sang from their hymnal. Next, the pale young lady with long, jet-black hair next to me chose a song no one had heard before. She must have been one of the last to arrive here since no one knew the artist or the song. The look on everyone's faces said it all when the choppy, incoherent video ended. We should be happy to be locked up in here if what was portrayed in the video reflected how far society had fallen. Everyone's eyes landed on me, the last in the room to choose.

"I used to like a song about honey from a rock. I don't know the name, though," I said, lifting my head to watch her scroll through videos. It didn't take her long to find a familiar thumbnail. "There, that's the one."

When the music started, a flood of sadness rushed over me. Wave after wave of memories crashed against my worn and tattered soul. I had a family once. A wife and two children. I knew where my wife was, but where were my children? They must have been taken up during the rapture. I couldn't remember having them at one point. God was protecting me from grief. As this new revelation consumed me, tears fell like a raging storm. My heart was smashed on the rocks and battered beyond repair. I had to go home, wherever home was now, but here it was not. Silence followed the song, and hand after hand landed on my back to console me. Tears raced down my cheeks, and the entire group surrounded me. Some were even praying.

The class was dismissed, and the teacher held the door open at the back of the room. She nodded with an empathetic smile as I walked past her. Ma saved me a chair at the closest seating area. Without much energy left, it looked inviting, even though I didn't want to socialize. Maybe they'd let me sit in silence for a while. The small group was quiet, enjoying the sun pouring through the skylight above us. Squeaks held her tongue much longer than I expected. Looking like a shaken can of root beer, her eyes gave away the pressure building without being able to talk. Unable to hold any longer, she left for a livelier bunch across the room.

Facing the laundry room door, I noticed a small, green half-circle below the knob that said *vacant*. I'd seen those before on restroom doors, and when locked from the inside, it turns into a red-occupied label. None of the other closed doors had locks. Not the classroom door, the bedroom doors, not even the doctor's door. "Why does the laundry room door have a lock like that?" I asked, looking at Ma and the preacher.

"To keep people out," said the preacher.

"Or in," said Marge from behind me. "I'm sure you were taken in there and not so pleasantly searched when you got checked in. Weren't you?"

"Yes." I nodded.

"Now imagine being a young, attractive female, doped up on meds and taken in there. It's not near as pleasant as your unpleasant experience. I can promise you that. Even when they halfway remember what happened the next day, between the meds and the darkness it's impossible to recognize or remember who did it. Who are they going to tell anyway? Have you noticed the staff aren't friendly? Helps to be an ugly old broad like me sometimes," she laughed, adjusting her glasses.

The room cleared for another smoke break, giving me time to recharge. While everyone was outside, a young, frizzy-haired blonde girl was escorted through the doors and left alone. She had been in the room next to me when my wife left. Her younger sister must have been taken in the rapture, leaving her to fend for herself here. Alone and frantic, she curled into a tight ball on a chair in the corner. Her hair hid most of her tiny frame, and she disappeared against the wall. The place was filled with noise and people when the smoke break finished. Her camouflage worked as intended, and no one noticed.

She was too young to be locked in with adults, so I sat in a not-so-distant chair to stand guard. After the stories about the staff, and not to mention the evil spirits con-trolling the people around here like puppets, she needed a protector. For the next hour, she remained a statue. To my relief, not a single person, inmate, or staff acknowledged she was in the room.

As the lunch line formed along the wall, she still didn't budge. I knelt at her chair and gently tapped her arm, not wanting to startle her. Telling her it was time to eat, she remained motionless.

Nudging her elbow with more effort, I told her, "Come on, it's safe. It's time to eat, and some friendly people are waiting for us." But nothing, no movement.

Her hair sprang back with a second tap on her arm as her head flew against the wall, and I fell backward. Two black pits were staring back from her tilted face. A single stream of blood ran down each cheek from the gaping holes. Straps the size of leather shoelaces bound her lips, preventing her from screaming. She panicked, but she couldn't break free. Her arms were cinched together by a white cotton rope.

I ran to the counter where one of the female staff was typing away. "She needs help. You have to help her," I pleaded.

"Help who?" she asked, jumping to her feet.

"The girl in the corner, she's all tied up and bleeding."

"What girl? Where?

"She's right there in the chair. See? Blonde frizzy hair?"

"Sir, there's no one over there. Look," she said, pointing at the wall.

"She's right—" The girl was gone. "She had to be somewhere. She can't be far. She's hurt. You have to find her."

"Sir, calm down. Here, you go with the others to lunch while I look for her. Maybe she's scared of all the people. I'll find her. Trust me. You go on now," she said, shooing me toward the lunch line, which was disappearing through the door.

Unable to eat, her face was burnt in my mind. People talked, ate, and laughed, but they didn't see her. How did they not see her? Why did no one help her? I sat on the cold tile by the door, hoping they found her, wanting to be the first out.

We returned to the common area after what seemed like forever, and she was nowhere to be found. Neither the girl nor the lady behind the counter. She must have left with her to get help. What a relief. I thought I could finally rest a minute, but the wooden doors bursting open killed my chance. A male physician pushing a small screen on a stick strutted in. He danced through the room, covered in red hearts, from his scrubs to his hair cover. "That's Dr. Love," said Marge. "Can you tell why?" She laughed.

"He doesn't seem like the good kind of love."

"Oh, he's not. He's one of the ones you need to look out for. He's a sleazeball."

"Whose room did he walk into?"

"He's in Squeak's room. You might walk by and check on her."

Taking her advice, I walked to Squeak's room and leaned on the door frame. Dr. Love's back was to me. Squeaks was sitting at the edge of the bed, feet dangling halfway to the floor. In true fashion, she was rambling a million miles a minute, but I never heard anyone talking back. Taking one soft step at a time into the room, the angle changed enough to see a blank screen. Squeaks was talking to her reflection as the doctor recorded her with his phone.

"Hey. Who's she supposed to be talking to?" I asked,

causing him to fumble his phone as Squeaks giggled.

"Her nutritionist, that's who," he responded. "You're not supposed to be in here. You need to get out."

"And she's not supposed to be talking to a blank screen either, but here we are."

"Her nutritionist just got off the line. Come on now. It's time for you to leave."

"I'm leaving when you're leaving. You good with me hanging out, Squeaks?"

"Oh, goody! Of course, you can!" she shouted, jumping from the bed and dancing.

"I'm done here anyway," said Dr. Love, shaking his head. "After you."

The doctor followed me out of her room, not strutting like before. I was standing by the door with my arms crossed as he emerged.

"What?" he barked.

"Waiting on you to see where we go next. This is fun. Put me in one of your videos, doc." The room went silent as he hung his head and rolled the little screen back to where he came from as fast as possible.

CHAPTER 15

Mary Lou and Jesse filled the open seats beside me. "My work here is done; time for me to go," I said, interrupting their conversation.

"But you can't go," said Mary Lou, straightening her posture. "There are hundreds of people waiting downstairs. Not many make it to where we're at. We're the lucky ones. If you go, someone else will take your spot. It's not easy to get in here."

The rapture. I hadn't thought about what life was like beyond the walls. No house to go home to. Life as I knew it had washed away while I had been here. *How complicated things must be without me right now.* I had heard my wife's voice on the phone but didn't know if my kids were safe. Or if they were still here on earth. "I need to find my family," I said, jumping to my feet.

I flew in for a crash landing and startled the new face at the counter. "Can I help you?" asked an angelic voice.

"I'd like to go home now. I need to call my wife."

"Let me check your file. Hold on one second," she said, walking to a silver file cabinet. "Your doctor hasn't said you can go yet. You should probably stay with us a little while longer."

"Ask the doctor. He'll tell you I'm fine."

"Okay," she said, punching the keys on the phone as she walked away. She returned a few minutes later, but her bright eyes had been replaced by a heaviness. "The doctor said you're well enough to go if you want, but I think you should stay with us for a few more days. Your new friends are going to miss you."

"My friends will be fine. Let me call my wife now."

A second staff member typing away at a nearby desk looked up and said, "All you need is a witness if he's going to check himself out." My guardian angel passed the phone.

Dialing the only set of numbers I still remembered, the excitement boiled over. Ring after ring was interrupted when her familiar voice on the other end said, "Hello."

"Hi, honey! The doctor said I'm good to go now. Will you come get me?"

"No. I'm not coming to get you. You need to stay there for at least seven days and take your medicine. You've been there two. You have to stay," she said.

"But the doctor said I'm fine and ready to go."

"Please stay there. I'm begging you. You have to take the medication and get some sleep."

"I'm not taking pills from these people. I don't trust them. It's time for me to go. I'm not staying."

"Please stay in there a little while longer. I'm begging you," she said.

"It's time for me to go, honey. I've already signed the papers, and I'm checking out now. Bye!"

Hanging up the phone, I asked the lady what was next. She said it might be a while before the papers were processed, but then I'd be free to go. Our conversation was interrupted by a tap on her shoulder. "Phone is for you," said the lady beside her.

"Yes, ma'am. The doctor said he was well enough to go home.... I understand you don't think he's okay to go home.... Ma'am, there's nothing we can do. He's already checked himself out.... The dismissal papers are in line to be signed by the doctor. He'll be let out the front door as soon as they're signed.... I understand, but legally there is nothing we can do.... Look, take him home, and call the cops when you arrive. Tell them you're scared, and he's getting violent. They'll pick him up and take him to the psych ward at the hospital. It's your only shot at admitting him where he can't check out on his own.... Yes, ma'am. I'll try and stall until you get here."

She hung up the phone and was surprised to see me when she turned back around.

"Soooo, when can I leave?"

"Have a seat over there, and I'll come to get you when it's time," she said with a smile as the angelic voice returned.

What seemed like hours of staring at the exit doors leading to freedom finally ended with a light tap on the shoulder. The doors I'd jiggled, pushed, and leaned into a hundred times opened like magic as we walked through. Pressure built like a kinked garden hose with each step down the narrow hall, exploding as we entered the main waiting room. There she was. My wife had made it. I hadn't been sure how I would find her on my own, but I knew God would provide, and there she was.

"Where's your bag?" she asked.

"What bag?"

"You're wearing the same clothes I dropped you off in. I packed you a bag, where is it?"

"Here's one behind the counter. We didn't know whose it was," said the receptionist holding a black backpack.

I sailed through the glass entry doors, breathing in the freedom. The air was fresh and clean, and flowers still weaved around the feet of the massive columns. The clear blue sky towered above, and the sun's warm kiss greeted my face. Not at all what I thought the earth would look like after the rapture, but I was glad it was still intact. Storming past me to the car, my wife led the way as I tried to wrap my brain around how beautiful the world remained.

"Why didn't you stay?" she cried out in frustration.

"It's okay. The doctor said I was fine."

"You're not fine. You shouldn't have checked yourself out. Where were you going to go if I hadn't got here?

You didn't even take any medication, not once," she said as her hands trembled with a lethal blend of frustration and anxiety.

I wasn't expecting this kind of reaction, but I didn't make it a habit to question God or my wife. "Did you see how vibrant and colorful the flowers were?" I asked in hopes of changing the subject.

Not wanting to discuss how lovely the landscaping was, she continued to grind on the self-approved early release. I, however, turned silent in anticipation of where we were going once the car was put in gear.

The roads were still jam-packed with cars and trucks, and life appeared to be moving forward seamlessly. Not as many people were taken up in the rapture as I expected. Not at first glance, anyway. The streets looked familiar as we pulled into a drive-through pharmacy. "What are we doing here?" I asked.

"We're picking up your medicine, and you will be taking it."

Through the speaker chimed the same angelic voice I had heard flow from the nurse upon checkout. My guardian angel was following me home. Her voice assured me that whatever came through the tiny box would be safe. We pulled out and drove toward where home used to be. Turning on the main drag, then into our neighborhood, my nerves burst like pop rocks. Our street still looked the same. There at the end, our house stood firm.

The garage door closed behind us, and we passed over the threshold to the mudroom. Our kids met us there with smiles and open arms. A wave of joy crashed over me. They were still here, and we were still a family. Even our yapping dog, Cooper, was ecstatic to see me. After the hugs, I turned my attention to the little furball. He flipped on his back for a belly rub, and as I leaned in, his eyes caught my spirit. Glowing back were the eyes of my guardian angel, telling me everything would be all right now.

My wife handed me three pills and a bottle of water. At first, I questioned why so many, but then I remembered I was safe at home, and I could trust her. Twenty-four hours later, my eyes opened to the fan blades spinning above my head. A few groggy hours of consciousness brought more pills and more sleep. The day after brought the first trip to the psychiatrist.

My brain was in a fog from the medication, and I

hadn't yet learned the fogginess was also my brain trying to wind down the rpms from running on red for days on end. I answered what questions I could, and by the time we left, my wife was relieved to hear a diagnosis. She would get her husband back. It was treatable. The ER doctor days prior hadn't done her any favors when he told her I would never be the same or work again most likely. I can't imagine the turmoil she experienced, having me ripped from reality right in front of her. I was still weeding the garden of my mind, searching for what didn't belong, so it was hard to follow the psychiatrist's conversation with my wife. While scheduling the follow-up, I saw the last flash of demonic eyes as the secretary confirmed my next appointment time.

Breaking through the vicious cycle of pills and sleep, I finally had an incredible yet grounding day. Two of my closest work friends stopped by to bring lunch and say hello. Later the same day, two more friends, whom I consider family, stopped by to see how I was doing. Smiling, I tried to hide the fact I didn't quite understand what happened, what was happening, and what would happen in the coming weeks. After their visit, when it was time for more pills and sleep, I asked my wife how long it had been since I'd gone to work. Her answer of three weeks sucker punched my fragile sense of reality.

As much as I missed work, I knew I wasn't ready to go back. My short-term memory flickered like a fluorescent bulb in an empty room. I was forgetting simple things like what I had done that day, and I misplaced items all over the house and outside. The first time I attempted to drive had me white-knuckled and regretting the decision. There was a terrifying delay from the time I knew the light had turned red to when my foot received the message to press the brake pedal. I couldn't get home soon enough.

The following weeks added to the longest span I had gone without working in my adult life. Filling the time with "normal" things to keep busy, I attempted to process what had happened. I struggled to decipher what was real, even though every bit was real to me. In turn, I questioned everything, attempting to find solid ground again.

Who defines real anyway? Was the combination of hallucinations and delusions the absolute truth of my experience? Were brain chemicals and environmental conditions truly responsible for launching me into an alternate reality that only existed in the theater of my mind? Or was there a chance spiritual warfare had played a role in what the natural world considered my psychotic break?

Lithium was the first long-term prescription given as I weaned off the stronger anti-psychotic sleep medication. This little pink pill for treating my newfound condition was the gold standard, or so I was told. It became the small thorn that will forever pierce my side twice a day, morning and night. For me, a daily reminder of what most considered everyday life was now a direct result of not forgetting to take the pills. The pills are the ceiling preventing my mind from reaching the heavens again and the chains holding my thoughts from wandering far away. Even with the medication, there is no guarantee it won't happen again. Even when clouds obscure the moon, it remains in the sky. Patiently waiting in the background for a tiny crack to gain a foothold and burst forth again.

The day came when I was cleared to return to work. Full of excitement, I felt truly blessed to have a work family who welcomed me back with open arms. The first few days were great at the surface level. Hugs, smiles, and friendly faces were the framework for easing back into a new daily routine. My old routine had been picked up and carried on in my absence. It was no longer mine to carry. It's funny how life works. Most people would love to do less or have it easier and still receive a paycheck. I, on the other hand, was filled with insecurity. I was unsure of who I was and where I fit in moving forward.

My mind and thought process were different after the psychotic break. I questioned if it was the medication or if my mind had been damaged, but there was no way of knowing for sure. More than likely, it was a little of both. Putting on a smile for others is hard when you don't even recognize yourself.

In the following days and weeks, I barely reached the front door before passing out from exhaustion. My brain no longer functioned at the level it used to. If I were to guess, operating at half what it used to would be a generous statement. The internet was kind enough to inform me that fatigue was one of lithium's many side effects, along with nonexistent short-term memory and slurred speech. My mouth moved faster than my brain could function. Inserting words that made no sense midsentence or twisting my tongue in such a manner that it stopped working altogether. The only consistent brain function I'd retained was replaying the psychedelic roller coaster of my psychosis every night when I closed my strained eyes. It was branded in my mind as the experience played like a looping movie.

I always thought depression was about being sad or a lack of motivation. Avoidable or reversible depending on one's character and willpower. My uninformed stance for years on the subject became glaring proof of my ignorance. To my surprise, sadness or any small remnant of a stray feeling would have been a welcome relief compared to the void left by depression.

It stole every ounce of emotion I had ever known, leaving nothing in its wake. No joy, no sadness, no hope, nothing. Words cannot describe the depth of emptiness the bottomless pit of depression leaves behind. With surgical precision, the very essence of life was carved from my being, and I was none the wiser as it happened. I now understood why in the Bible people close to Jesus longed for death after he ascended. My connection to this world was withered and dying, and my separation from God felt worse than death itself.

Watching me suffer, my wife broke through the darkness and scheduled another appointment with the psychiatrist. Describing my days, moods, exhaustion, and foggy brain, he found it best to prescribe an antidepressant. I was the guy who never took medicine for anything. No doctors, no meds, and I had never been depressed for a day in my life. Or so I thought. Turns out depression is a thief with many faces. What was one more pill, right?

After a few short days, the color returned to life. Energy, smiling, and laughter—real heartfelt laughter—returned. I had no idea how deep depression had pulled me down its dark and empty pit until I saw the sunshine again like it was the first time. But as the weeks marched on, the antidepressant wasn't strong enough to keep the beast at bay. Happiness was pulled away like the frayed ends of a rope. Taking little pieces until I was left with nothing again. Pride may be a warrior, but from my experience, his sword is always pointed in the wrong direction. Seeing this, my wife stepped in and called the psychiatrist for me. I wasn't surprised when his name appeared on my phone. Agreeing to up the antidepressant dosage, we hung up.

Almost a year removed, I considered myself one of the

lucky ones for many reasons after circling the mountain with God. I had also been wrestling with emotions that constantly bounced between a drug-induced floor and ceiling. Never too high, never too low, but continually changing. Before this, I went forty years without any significant life-altering events. On the backside, my medications were lined out in a relatively quick fashion compared to most. I had not only friends and family praying for me but strangers as well. People whom I'd never met and probably never would were lifting me up in prayer for recovery. I was surrounded by a loving family and loving friends. I even returned to work surrounded by nothing but support and love from my work family.

My experience was a flash in the pan compared to what others have experienced. They spend years trying medication after medication, doctor after doctor, fighting for their lives. Some have been stuck in the storm their whole lives with no love, no support, and no prayers to speak of. Hanging on by a tiny thread. Others don't survive the storm. The drive to someday help pull people back from the darkness keeps me going. God put it on my heart to create a bridge of understanding between those who suffer and those who have never seen the pain below the surface of a hurting smile. The constant ringing in my ears, stiff muscles, fatigue, and a malfunctioning thyroid from medication is a small price to pay compared to some. I am truly blessed.

I know God created the heavens, the earth, and everything in between, and I also know He was and will forever be in control, beginning to end. Even so, I can't help but wonder why He took me to the edge of insanity and back.

CHAPTER 16

From my experience with psychosis, I have concluded that normal is relative to the reality in which you are accustomed. Walking through psychosis amid delusions and hallucinations seemed perfectly normal while it was happening. As my spirit moved through space and time, I was a passenger who knew no different. I heard every sound and smelled every smell with an intensity I had never dreamed possible. My eyes were microscopes, enhancing the world's depth and detail. It even saddens me to know most people will never fathom the world as I experienced. So full of beauty and life it was hard to return to what most perceive as real. Time no longer existed where I was. No deadlines to meet or places to be. I could smell the tiniest flowers from ten feet away as they radiated every color of the rainbow. Even a slight breeze caressed my entire body like a silk sheet.

If my wife or I had known lack of sleep was one of the first signs of mania, it would have made no difference. She was sound asleep, and I enjoyed the extra hours added to my day, with the exception of when I thought our home was under siege. The sleepless string of nights leading up to the psychiatric hospital set the stage for the climax of my psychosis. Looking back, I'm grateful. Had I not been in psychosis, I would not have prayed with or spoken to the people I encountered. I would have been cowering in a corner, hoping no one noticed me, scared to death. Did any of my conversations or prayers make a difference in anyone's life? Who knows, but I'd like to think they did. Remembering what took place over those few weeks seared my brain like a cattle brand, but deciphering the difference between reality, delusions, and hallucinations is a different kind of pill to swallow, pun intended.

If a parent abandoned a child or someone's spouse left them, they would have difficulty trusting again. In both situations, a lack of trust would be understandable, even expected in most cases. I never imagined that waking up one morning and no longer trusting my own mind or thoughts could be a reality. Rising early, alert, and ready to conquer the day is something most people long for. That is no longer the case for me, however. An energetic start to the day releases an irrational flood of alarms. Am I manic? Did I forget the lithium? Have my imbalanced brain chemicals finally overpowered the little pink pills? If I go manic, would I know it this time, or would I make a fool of myself? I've heard rumbling tracks beneath my feet would mean nothing if I'd never seen a train. I'm hopeful that's the case considering I rode the last one all the way to the scene of the crash before knowing what it was.

The alternative to energetic mornings finds me more often, like most people. Slow to rise and get moving before a shower and a cup of caffeine-free coffee. This typical morning for most still causes an obscene sense of concern for me some days, and I question everything. I suppose that's why it's called bipolar. Is this a normal tiredness, or is the antidepressant not strong enough anymore? It could be my thyroid again, because I was exhausted when those levels got out of whack. Or could it be depression was back, clawing at my feet, trying to finish the job?

Either start to the day must be wrestled down and subdued before any personal interactions occur. Looking happier than usual might send up a red flag, but heavy eyes are sure to provoke my least favorite question, the dreaded, "Is everything okay?" I don't know how to answer it, considering I had no idea the last time when I wasn't. From my experience, most people want to know how you're doing until you give them a real answer. Not that they're to blame, because I don't want to give an honest answer as much, if not more, than they want to receive it. It takes practice to find the sweet spot, smack dab in the middle, to blend with the crowd.

These are some things I've wrestled with over the year following my psychosis. Spending many days and nights hiding in the dark corners of my mind. Getting caught up and lost in how the world defines mental illness is like quicksand. Better yet, how it defines people with a mental illness. These definitions often come in one of three forms: lies, facts, or truth.

Lies can lead to destruction if allowed to grow roots. They wear many faces and come from many places. The worst are the lies I can tell myself. These lies say I'll never be the same again. I'm broken, damaged, and worthless to those around me. Why bother rebuilding? There's no hope for the future. Getting out of bed is pointless. It will happen again, and next time will be way worse. I'll pass this on to my kids, and their lives will be ruined. These lies smirk in the background when I'm happy, waiting for a misstep so they can say, "I told you so." They sneak in at any opportunity and create debilitating fear, destroying any sense of worth and well-being if allowed. They make a room full of people feel like the loneliest place in the world because no one understands. These lies, among many more, crush and steal countless lives daily.

As a Christian, I've also heard a staggering arsenal of lies attacking the salvation and faith of those living with mental illness. Things like medication wouldn't be needed if I really believed in God. Or mental illness is demonic possession. A good friend once told me he believed God healed in three ways, and I tend to agree with him, though there are probably many more. Those three ways are healing through miracles, over time, and by medication.

The more time I put between myself and the psychotic break, the more I am at peace. With time comes acceptance and understanding. I have learned to accept the things I still do not understand because God was in control then, the same as He is now. In regard to miracles, John 14:12 says, "Very truly I tell you, whoever believes in me will do the works I have been doing, and they will do even greater things than these because I am going to the Father" (NIV).

Jesus said those who believe in him will do even greater works. This includes miracles. Miracles still happen today, every day, to be exact. All the modern technology, techniques, and medications that save and prolong lives are a small portion of those miracles. God blessed many different people in different ways to produce all of these. When people have allergies, they take allergy medication. Aspirin for temporary headaches and medications for high cholesterol and blood pressure are all taken without a second thought. Mental illness carries a different stigma, even though the brain is the most challenging and complex organ in the body to understand. If medications are suitable for healing other ailments and improving bodily functions, why is mental illness viewed differently? I will never understand the double standard, but my hope is to open the door for conversation and understanding.

Then there are facts. Facts are what the world says bipolar is and what I should expect from here on out. When searching for answers, these facts fall out of life's magic little eight-ball called the internet. They say bipolar is a severe mental illness, an incurable disease, and is one of the leading causes of disability in the world. The facts also say bipolar reduces life expectancy by nine to ten years, depending on which factual report populates the screen. One of the main reasons for this haunting fact is about forty percent of people with bipolar disorder attempt suicide, and one in five are successful. Add in the mix that around fifty percent of marriages fail when one of the partners has bipolar. Not to mention most medications come with a laundry list of side effects. Facts may be facts, but sometimes they are no more pleasant than lies.

The key is to flip the factual coin to the positive side. This side of the coin says there is a bountiful list of successful artists, writers, musicians, actors, and actresses who wake up daily living with bipolar. Some of the world's most prolific minds are fueled by what some call a disease, illness, or disorder. I don't believe this is an accident. More like they found their calling by using their gifts as God intended. There are also countless people succeeding in life who have bipolar and spend their time pushing forward unnoticed unless they were to bring attention to it. The fact is that every day is layered with choices that directly affect the outcome. Happily ever after is never a fairytale ending. It's a choice to love myself and others exactly where I am in the pursuit of truth.

The truth is who God says I am and His promise of who I can become. God is our creator, and He created us in His image, so I don't find it a coincidence that people with bipolar disorder are most known for being creative. I find it a blessing. God doesn't make mistakes. This is sometimes hard to wrestle with, but it's a truth, none-theless. Therefore, since I believe God is my creator and doesn't make mistakes, I have been created for such a time as this. It's now my job to find out how I am supposed to use my time, talents, and experiences to be a blessing and help as many people as possible. Ephesians 2:10 says, "For we are God's handiwork, created in Christ Jesus to do good works, which God prepared in advance for us to do" (NIV). I fully intend to step into my pre-appointed purpose as God reveals it. This is the truth I find comfort in.

Another truth is the sheer strength it takes to not only accept having a mental illness but having the ability to subdue it and live a successful life. My vision of strength was entirely wrong before walking through psychosis and the healing process on the backside. I have learned it takes more strength to not hold in the hurt and confusion. It's not easy to ask for help, to admit I don't have it all together. I was raised to take it on the chin and keep it moving, but suffering in silence isn't strength, nor is it sustainable. Being vulnerable around family and friends has been the most challenging adjustment. I wouldn't be where I'm at without all of them. I had to get comfortable with the truth that doing my best looks different every day, and that's okay.

Truth comes under fire not only from lies and facts but also from feelings. Through reflection, I have learned my faith has to be stronger than my feelings, or I'll live the rest of my life thinking I'm a failure. Most people confuse feelings with emotions. Emotions are instinctual for all humans, bubbling up from the subconscious and existing independently of feelings. Joy, sadness, fear, anger, and anticipation are emotions, to name a few. They are as much a part of us as our personality and contribute to who we are.

On the other hand, feelings are learned responses to emotional triggers and are often irrational and vague. Feelings can cause more harm internally to an individual than other people ever could. In my own experience, since being diagnosed with bipolar, feelings have exploded in intensity and are much harder to contain. It's easy to get lost in things like feeling alone in a group of people. Feeling like not getting out of bed or going to work. Feeling like no one understands. Feeling lost and afraid. Feelings don't discriminate, nor do they care what time of day it is or what plans they're disrupting.

The good news is that every time feelings show up to take over, a choice must be made to let them control me or to subdue them. There is no in-between. Sometimes, it's okay to not be okay, but staying there too long isn't good for anyone. For every lie feelings try to convince me of, there are many truths in the Bible to keep me on the right path. Instead of fear, I'll take 2 Timothy 1:7 any day. It says, "For the Spirit God gave us does not make us timid, but gives us power, love, and discipline" (NIV).

While I do not understand why I'm now living with bipolar, I find comfort in the promises of God for my future. Three of my favorite promises in the Bible, ones I hang my hat on, are in John 9:1-4, where Jesus was walking with his disciples. We read, "As he went along, he saw a man blind from birth. His disciples asked him, 'Rabbi, who sinned, this man or his parents, that he was born blind?' 'Neither this man nor his parents sinned,' said Jesus, 'but this happened so that the works of God might be displayed in him. As long as it is day, we must do the works of him who sent me. Night is coming, when no one can work'" (NIV). Jesus then spits in the dirt, rubs mud in the blind man's eyes, and tells him to get up and go wash them out.

There is a lot to unpack from those verses, and they may have a different impact on different people, which is why it's called the Living Word. These verses tell me that even though Bipolar 1 is considered a severe mental illness, it is not some form of cosmic punishment for something my parents or I have done. This may sound weird to those who have never experienced the condescending spirit of religion, but trust me, it happens. Religion and

Christianity are two very different things. Jesus had to tell his disciples, who spent every waking moment with him, that the man wasn't blind because of sin. The second promise these verses tell me is I now have a mission to display God's work through me. To help people find faith, to give people hope, and to show people love who might otherwise never experience what God has to offer. Jesus said the man was blind so the works of God would be displayed through him. The last promise truly inspires me, and most people miss it altogether. The blind man was still blind when Jesus told him to get up and walk to the Pool of Siloam. He could have been healed instantly, so why was he told to stand and walk? The blind man had to walk by faith before he could experience the miracle. I have learned that sometimes you must walk through the darkness, not knowing why, before experiencing the blessing on the other side.

Even though no one knows what tomorrow holds, it's easier to face it with a circle of family and friends. There were many times I tried to shut people out during my healing process. On more than one occasion I broke harder than I ever had before, erupting in uncontrollable tears.

It was like all the emotions I had bottled up my entire life burst forth in a single moment. My wife was there to hold me tight even as I pushed her away. She wouldn't let go.

I wish I could give some quick, earth-shattering revelation to family members or friends of someone who suffers from mental illness. Or even an easy ten-step guide to follow, but the truth is, there is no such thing. A diagnosis is the first step in a lifelong journey for not only the individual but their family and friends as well. The best advice I can give to everyone involved is to never give up.

If this book ever lands in the hands of someone suffering in silence, I want you to know you are not alone. It is okay to not understand why or how it reached this point, and the main thing is you're still here. Many people didn't make it through yesterday, but you did. Isaiah 9:2 says, "The people walking in darkness have seen a great light; on those living in the land of deep darkness a light has dawned" (NIV). Today can be the first day of the rest of your life. The past can't be undone, but today is what you make it. People are suffering right now that only you can reach because of who you are and what you've been through. They need a community of support the same as we do. The truth is that the meaning of our lives isn't about what our lives mean to us. It's about what our lives mean to those around us. Not just family and friends but also those we reach out to when no one else will. Telling your own story will inspire hope in others and provide healing for you.

I want to thank all those who stood by me on this journey, and I hope they can someday pardon my psychosis.

| The End |

FAMILY RESOURCES

If you or someone you love needs help associated with a mental illness and aren't sure where to turn, I've compiled the list below as a starting point.

The first and best place to start is with in-person mental health assistance. While blog posts and videos from the internet may be a good resource, they will never take the place of individualized health care. Nor do they replace a good support system comprised of family and friends. Every person is unique, and treatment should be as well.

There's a long list of professionals who can help navigate a mental illness. Start with a diagnosis from a doctor or psychiatrist. Most of the time, they work closely together to determine a diagnosis as well as what medication will work best for the individual.

After a diagnosis, there are social workers, therapists, counselors, support groups, and faith groups for further support. A support system is a huge resource in navigating a mental illness diagnosis. No one should navigate life or a mental illness alone.

No matter how alone you may feel, please know there are people out there who care about you and want to help. Don't suffer in silence, and don't give up. It gets better, but remember, no one can help if you don't reach out.

Dial 988 or dial 911 in a life-threatening situation. The US Crisis Lifeline can be found at 988lifeline.org.

Findtreatment.gov is a website that can assist in finding a good treatment facility.

The American Psychiatry Association has a directory at Psychiatry.org for finding local psychiatrists.

The National Alliance on Mental Illness boasts 600 state organizations and affiliates. There's a good chance they have someone locally who can help. They can be found at Nami.org.

BOOK CLUB QUESTIONS

CH 1

In chapter one, the author poses this series of questions: *Was the combination of hallucinations and delusions the absolute truth of my experience? Were brain chemicals and environmental conditions truly responsible for launching me into an alternate reality that only existed in the theater of my mind? Or was there a chance spiritual warfare played a role in what the natural world considered my psychotic break?* What are your thoughts on the causes of mental illness?

How has our culture shaped your opinion of mental illness? Have any movies or television shows influenced how you view bipolar disorder?

Would you know the signs of mania if they presented in a friend or family member? If yes, how so? If not, how might it benefit you to know them?

CH 2

In chapter two, what do you think James's coworkers thought when he announced they were supposed to build a modern-day ark? How would you have reacted? Do you think someone should have caught on by then that something wasn't right? Why or why not?

How would you react to Death himself waltzing around your bedroom? Would you have jumped up and gone after him, or frozen like the author? Why?

CH 3

Do you think the truck blaring its horn and the dashboard light show was an electrical issue, a hallucination, or a spiritual attack?

James experiences visual, auditory, and olfactory hallucinations in chapter three. Can you find an example of each in the chapter?

CH 4

In chapter four, can you name some events that most likely happened and compare them to some you believe only occurred in his mind? What made you come to those conclusions?

James's watch quit working during his lunch outing. Do you think it was a coincidence? Discuss why or why not.

CH 5

Did this chapter do a good job of displaying the vast difference between what's going on in a manic mind versus what other people are experiencing? Which scene showed the most contrast, in your opinion?

James speaks of balance several times; do you think it is subconsciously connected to his mind being out of balance?

At what point in this chapter would you question what was happening if you were his coworker? What action would you have taken and why? If you have been diagnosed with a mental illness, how would you want coworkers to react in a similar situation?

CH 6

If you realized a coworker you cared about was breaking down like James at the beginning of this chapter, what would you do to help? What if they didn't know they needed help and refused? Do you think his coworkers did a good job of trying to help?

What would you do if you came home to your spouse baptizing themselves in the pool when they were supposed to be at work?

CH 7

How do you feel about hospitals? Can you imagine living through the description given of the emergency room waiting area? How would you have reacted?

How would you have reacted to the emergency room doctor if given the same inconclusive results? Have you ever left a hospital or doctor's office with more questions than when you arrived? What was your reaction?

CH 8

Have you ever taken time to enjoy nature or the sunrise, as James does in the open scene of this chapter? Do you think there were actual crows in the trees, or were they all hallucinations? What difference does this make to the way you read the story?

What scene stood out most in this chapter and why?

CH 9

If you put yourself in the shoes of James's wife, what emotions would you be wrestling with about the decision to drop your spouse off at a psychiatric hospital?

Which scene stands out the most as a hallucination? Which one stands out the most as a delusion?

CH 10

James's wife had her mother there for support. Who would you call for support if you had to admit your spouse or a loved one to a psychiatric hospital?

What would your first few hours be like if you were admitted to an inpatient psychiatric hospital? Would you act differently than James or similarly?

CH 11

This chapter starts in the morning, with patients congregating in the common area. Would you try to make friends, hide in your room, or wait until someone spoke to you first? Why?

Which person in this chapter stands out the most to you and why?

How would you have reacted to getting barged in on while preparing to shower?

CH 12

Do you think the lady in the cross T-shirt was delusional, or do you think one of the girls she rescued showed up in the psychiatric hospital with them?

Why do you think the therapist was shaking? Would you be nervous leading a group behind closed doors in a small room with psychiatric patients? Why do you think someone would want to work there?

Would you have kicked James out of the group therapy session as well? Why or why not?

CH 13

In this chapter, James speaks to a lady Ma claims to be a witch. Would you have approached her for a conversation or steered clear? Do you think there's a chance she was an ordinary lady, and Ma knew James had been hallucinating, so she made it up for pure entertainment?

Do you believe the young couple was sent in by an organization to report human trafficking, or were they making it up?

CH 14

Do you think James's conversation with Jesse and the hallucination about her had anything to do with divine intervention, or was it only by chance that they spoke the night before?

Was Nia speaking a different language, or were the people surrounding them delusional and only thought she was? Do you think there's a chance the other patients were only messing with James because they knew he was in psychosis?

CH 15

If your spouse checked themselves out of a psychiatric hospital, what is the first thing that would run through your mind? Would you follow the nurse's advice and call the cops so they would be admitted without the ability to check themselves out? Why or why not?

This chapter begins some of the initial healing and recovery. Do you believe healing and recovery were needed for both James and his wife? If so, how would it look different for each?

In this chapter, James details his first experience with depression. Have you or someone you know battled depression? How does that experience differ from James's?

CH 16

Reflecting on life-changing events can be healthy. Would James or his wife see psychosis coming if it happened again? Have any life-changing events snuck up on you? If so, what happened, and what was the outcome? Did you learn and grow from it?

This chapter explores the stigma surrounding faith and mental illness. If you are a Christian, what are your thoughts on this topic? If not, discuss the stigma surrounding mental illness in our current culture.

WRAP UP QUESTIONS

This book is a nonfiction memoir, but what genre would it fall under if it were fiction, and why?

Does the fact that James's reality while in psychosis was different than the world around him influence how "true" the memoir is, in your opinion?

What scene in the book left the biggest impression on you and why?

Have you or someone you know been diagnosed with a mental illness? If so, has this book changed your perspective in any way?

If you were to recommend this book to someone, who would it be and why?

ACKNOWLEDGMENTS

To say that I am truly blessed is an understatement. The amount of love and support I received from those around me during the events contained in this memoir and to this day has helped me heal and grow into the person I am today.

To my wife Julie, the definition of strength through the storm. Not only did you hold our family together during my psychosis, but you also held it together while bringing me back to reality. Without you, I wouldn't be who I am today, and I'll love you to the end of time and back.

To Katlyn, my wonderful daughter who is wise beyond her years. At such a young age, you realized all good things come from God and set a blazing trail for the rest of us to follow. Your drive and work ethic will take you anywhere you want to go, and you are wise enough to listen for where God wants to take you. You are my baby girl and a true blessing; I love you, sweetie.

To Jace, my amazing son, who is a much better and brighter version of myself. I'm truly blessed to be able to grow up alongside you. Lego set building, playing catch in the yard, and even the video games you ruthlessly beat me at are all a joy as you make each day brighter for me and all those around you. I can't wait to see the man you will grow into. I love you, buddy.

Dr Barnhart, I can't thank you enough for your expertise and guidance. I'm very blessed and grateful that you took me on as a patient, dialed in the medication I needed quickly, and have been there ever since. Thank you for helping me find the balance in my life again.

To my work family, who welcomed me back with open arms, not knowing what to expect or who I had become through my experience. Your kindness and support played a significant part in helping me walk through the most confusing time in my life. Without you, I would not be who I am today. I don't take that for granted because most people aren't as lucky. Thank you from the bottom of my heart.

To Tommy, you're like the older brother I never had, and I'm not referring to age. I'm talking about the sense of calm and peace you bring to any problem or situation life brings you. The overwhelming sense of security you bring makes everyone around you feel as if everything will be alright, and with you involved, everything will be. I'm truly blessed to call you a friend and consider you a brother.

Chad, I wouldn't be the person I am today without your guidance and mentorship. Your pursuit of wisdom through God's Word has kept me moving in the right direction in my own walk. Your ability to find good in every person and situation inspires those around you, especially me. I'm blessed to consider you a brother and call you my friend.

To Kevin, one of the best friends I could ask for. I know deep down you have a heart bigger than most. I will forever be grateful for how you handled my psychotic break and welcomed me back to work like we never skipped a beat. You have been a bigger part of my recovery than you'll ever know, and I'm blessed to have you in my life.

A thousand thanks to Eric F., the man who pushed me to spend time in God's presence, which led to writing this book. Thank you for reading my memoir and advising me through the process. You have coached me not only in my work life but also in my personal life; for that, I am forever grateful. I believe you were placed in my life at the perfect time, and the results will be plentiful throughout the rest of my life because of your impact.

To Chet T., a friend and mentor whom God brought into my life and has kept close through the years. Our coffee and lunch meetings have led to many great things in my life, including my salvation. Thank you for being a part of my family's lives.

I want to thank Kim and Mandy for investing the time to read this memoir and offer input long before it was released. I truly appreciate your time and input.

Author Photo credit goes to Brandon, my long-time and very dear friend.

Thank you to Caryn Rivadeneira for this manuscript's developmental and copy editing. I really appreciated your kind words and guidance through the process.

Special thanks to Trinity McFadden, who proofread the final manuscript.

I would also like to thank Rafael Andres for the cover design and formatting.

Psalm 30:1-4 (NIV)

I will exalt you, Lord,

For you lifted me out of the depths

And did not let my enemies gloat over me.

Lord my God, I called to you for help,

And you healed me.

You, Lord, brought me up from the realm of the dead;

You spared me from going down to the pit.

Sing the praises of the Lord, you his faithful people;

Praise his holy name.

www.jamescoast.com

www.voicelesstovictory.org